What is *Pono*?

"Pono is a concept worth adopting in our own life. If each of us really aspired to be pono, if we accepted our implicit agreement to be a pono spiritual being, a pono guardian of the earth's resources, a pono daughter or son, a pono spouse, friend, co-worker, employer, government servant — what a different world we could live in. I think it's a concept worth working for."

— Kumu Kea
Hawaiian Hula and
spirituality practitioner

"To put it very simply, living pono is living righteously, with a conscious decision to do the right thing in terms of self, others, and the environment."

— Rick Bacigalupi
Emmy Award-winner,
producer, "Toward Living Pono"

Green Living Ideas for Your Pono Home

bright ideas to reduce your
energy bills and live healthier

by Scott Cooney, MS, MBA

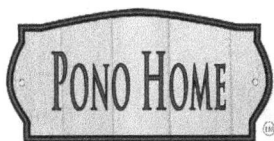

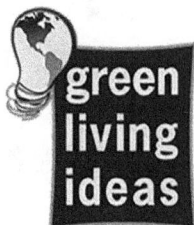

www.PonoHome.com
www.GreenLivingIdeas.com

To all those working to create a better world, whether it's the world around us or the world inside our own homes, I dedicate this book, love, and gratitude.

Acknowledgments

As sustainability gains widespread support and capitalizes on ever-improving disruptive technologies, one thing remains abundantly clear: bringing sustainability into the home is one of the greatest challenges we face. The *Green Living Ideas* initiative grew out of many conversations over many years with leading edge sustainability professionals. The fundamental underlying question: how do we make green living appealing enough to the masses to move the needle in global health, building sustainable, local, and self-reliant economies, and reducing global emissions?

The result of our work and collaboration with many of these professionals is now in your hands, and coming to your community soon, as Pono Home expands its maintenance and installation services to help make homes healthier and more efficient across the country and around the world. I would like to thank Jennifer Milholen for her dedicated focus on bringing these visions to reality. Her work and tireless commitment to making the world a better place were a key inspiration and testing ground for many of the concepts in the Pono Home service and in the pages of *Green Living Ideas*.

I also wish to express great gratitude to Peter Young, another dedicated sustainability professional working tirelessly to improve life on this planet for all its inhabitants, and Sara Cobble, who helped develop and design this book. Peter contributed substantial research and development time for *Green Living Ideas* while Sara brought a wonderful level of enthusiasm and positivity to help bring these efforts across the finish line.

Sarah DePhillips, a visionary creator in her own right, has

added innumerable advancements to our company and helped inform the direction and content in this book to be ever more helpful to those who are far along, as well as those who are just starting their sustainability journeys. Anthony Ng's fantastic work ethic combined with an impressive ability to get things done has advanced Pono Home beyond where I'd envisioned it could go in a shorter time frame than most anyone thought possible.

Members of the Important Media family (www.ImportantMedia.org) also contributed in many more ways than we can count to the creation of the concepts all the way through to fruition. Zach Shahan, Site Director for CleanTechnica, the world's largest clean tech news site with 5 million monthly readers, has helped create a global movement toward sustainability in the energy sector that transcends political boundaries and has shifted global markets in profound ways. Derek Markham has helped launch Important Media as a jack-of-all-trades with a penchant for finding just the right solution, and has helped me transition all of my energies to Pono Home after splitting time between the companies for a few years.

Our work would be years away without the assistance of the Hawaii-based Elemental Excelerator, a clean tech incubator that chose Pono Home to be part of its 2014 and 2016 cohorts of companies with the potential to wean Hawaii, and the world, off fossil fuels. With the help of the Excelerator, Pono Home was able to find its footing. At the time of this writing, our little company has now performed green retrofits in over 5,000 homes in Hawaii, many of them lower income, hard-to-reach, multilingual families that would otherwise not be exposed to sustainability through more traditional means.

To all of these people and many more that space and time

do not allow inclusion in these pages, I am forever grateful that you live the life Ghandi professed: to be the change you want to see in the world. Together, we'll make it all happen.

— Scott Cooney

Contents

Is Solar the Best Option to Green a Home?

For many people, the first thing they think about when considering greening their home is a home solar PV (photovoltaic) system. Home solar PV systems generate electricity from the sun that is used directly in your home, and can also be sent back into the electrical grid if there is excess created. In many cases, utilities will be required to pay homeowners for producing extra electricity and sending it into the grid, since they can sell it to a neighbor's home and make a markup on it. Sometimes utilities pay homeowners with solar systems that produce extra electricity in the form of cash, but sometimes it is simply credit toward future energy bills when the solar production is not as high as the demand in the home (common in winter, for instance).

Solar is, without a doubt, a wonderful thing for many people. It can be used quite effectively as far north as Alaska, and in countries as cloudy as Germany, where solar power generating capacity is now higher than any other form of power, according to a report published on CleanTechnica. com.[i]

Over the last 10 years, solar panels have dropped in price substantially, and have improved in performance markedly, making them a better investment than ever. Is solar right for your home? It's a complicated question with many variables. But if you want to do some research, Pono Home recommends visiting Cleantechnica,com for more information on solar:

http://cleantechnica.com/solar-power.

Other green upgrades

Solar is a big investment with a lot of moving parts. There are permits, contractors, roofing decisions, and long term planning. It's a wonderful investment for many people, and we highly encourage you to take that step. Financing options are typically available if you have reasonable credit, meaning you might pay nothing up front, and just pay for the solar system over time with the savings you're getting on your electric bill.

But there is so much more you can do that costs almost nothing, requires no permits, electrical work, or roofing contractors, and that's what we think should happen first and foremost. And that's the subject of the rest of this book. Energy and water efficiency are hands-down one of the best investments you'll ever make, and we hope you'll find thousands of dollars in savings over your lifetime with the simple steps outlined in Section I, as well as improving your health and the health of your family's home in Section II.

Further reading on solar:

Solar power
http://cleantechnica.com/solar-power/

Is a home solar PV system right for you?
http://homesolarpv.com/

Which solar panels are most efficient?
http://cleantechnica.com/2014/02/02/which-solar-panels-most-efficient/

How solar panels work
http://solarlove.org/how-solar-cells-work-components-op-eration-of-solar-cells/

Solar Energy Facts & Figures
http://solarlove.org/solar-energy-facts-solar-power-facts/

Introduction

What would you do with a hundred extra bucks a month? What if, rather than making that money by working harder than you already do, you make it by living better? What if you can get that hundred bucks without having to ask for a raise, without staying late at the office, or without spending less on eating out or shopping? Any financial counselor would tell you that reducing your spending is far better than getting a pay raise. It's what economists call "after-tax income" and it's much more valuable than "pre-tax income," which you have to pay taxes on before you can spend or save it.

Let's take it a step further. What if, rather than just for a month or a couple of months, you could get that money for the rest of your life? An extra $1,000 or so a year...a fun fantasy, right? Here's the thing: it's not a fantasy. Many of us spend far more money than we need to on our home utility bills and the gas we put into our car. In many cases, especially with the increasing cost of energy, this can add up to a few hundred dollars a month in wasted money.

Your money is your money. You shouldn't have to waste it just to live your day-to-day life. By making just a few small tweaks to your home, you can save hundreds, even thousands of dollars every year, for the rest of your life. This book will show you how.

According to a McKinsey & Company study, people in the U.S. could save $420 billion (that's $420,000,000,000.00) PER YEAR if their homes were more energy efficient.[ii]

$420 billion across the country seems like a lot, but what does that number really mean to you? Would that make much of a difference in your life? You bet. Consider this: a 2012 study of 71,000 homes in 38 states found that peoplewho buy energy efficient homes are 32% less likely to default than those who buy inefficient homes.[iii] When you consider everything that could factor into a default: losing a job, divorce, illness, accidents, pay cuts, lawsuits, tightening credit...isn't it amazing to think that utility costs can make that much of a difference?

Realistically, though, it's not that surprising. Calculating your mortgage payments, car payments, insurance payments, and other fixed costs is pretty straightforward, so it's easier to plan for. Calculating the average electricity, water, and sewer costs for a potential home you're buying is much less predictable. Your family will use that house much differently than the previous occupants, right? And when you have a life, a family, a job...who has the time or know-how to figure out where your electricity is being used, and whether there are savings to be had?

And what about renters? You can't just go and swap out your appliances for energy efficient models, and certainly you're not going to pony up a few thousand dollars to add some extra insulation to your attic, so it's out of your hands right? The good news is that, homeowner or renter, across the country and across the world, there are hundreds of billions of dollars of savings to be realized. We only need to make some small infrastructural and behavioral changes in how we understand and use energy and water. The even better news is that many of these changes can be done whether you're a long time homeowner or a short-term renter, and the return on investment starts from DAY ONE.

While we're at it, why not improve your health by removing some toxins from your home? Greener living is healthier living, after all.

No matter how "green" you are, your home is likely to be a hotbed of toxic stuff. Between the weed-n-feed in your garage, old paint cans in your basement, bug sprays under your sink, cleansers in your bathroom, and detergents in your laundry room, you more than likely have dozens, if not hundreds, of potentially carcinogenic chemicals lurking in your home. An unfortunate reality, but it can be fixed!

We are exposed to these chemicals in many ways. For instance, most people know that when you paint a room, you're supposed to let it air out for a few days by leaving the windows open. Why? What you may think of as a bad smell or something that may give you a headache is actually chemicals that escape the paint as it dries, a phenomenon known as "off-gassing." And it's not just fresh paint that contains chemicals. Many consumer products off-gas a bevy of airborne pollutants in your home. Conventional chemicals used in the manufacture of bed linens, furniture, pet beds, paints, plasters, and even kids' cribs routinely off-gas airborne pollutants. One prominent example is formaldehyde, a probable carcinogen, which will off-gas for many years, not just for the first few days.

Additionally, personal care products can routinely contain ingredients that are known, probable, and/or suspected carcinogens that you are ingesting and/or putting on your skin every day. You may not have known, but absorption through your skin can account for up to 90% of your total intake of chemicals from the environment.[iv]

Plus, you're eating it. Ingredients in your food that are regularly approved by the Food and Drug Administration have been implicated in everything from ADD/ADHD to nausea to chronic inflammation to allergies to cancer, and more! All of these chemicals may contribute to your body's chemical burden.

Had enough? We are here to make it better. This book is full of practical, easy to implement strategies and practices that can benefit both homeowners and renters by saving money, as well as reducing or even eliminating your exposure to toxins. Make habits of these practices, and you'll be on the road to healthier, wealthier living, for the rest of your life. Some would call it "sustainability". Others maybe "green living ideas." Call it what you will, the primary impact of these efforts is to make your life better.

So who are we to tell you this, and why should you believe us? For us, and people like us, sustainability is very personal. While I care deeply about the plight of the polar bears and the peoples of the Amazon rainforest that have had their livelihoods crushed by ruthless and greedy oil exploration and its toxic legacy, ultimately, sustainability for me was a choice I made for personal benefit. My life is better because I live sustainably. The socioeconomic benefits, the public health benefits, and the benefits to polar bears and icecaps are the icing on the cake that make this lifestyle so gratifying.

"Living green" has saved me at least $100,000 in post-tax money in the last 20 years or so, and it has been great for my health.

At age 17, my doctor found that I had not escaped my family history of high cholesterol. My cholesterol reading was well over 300, and, in the prime physical condition of my life, my doctor recommended I go on a cholesterol reduction drug. Maybe you've noticed that pharmaceutical drugs are not cheap? Going on a cholesterol reduction drug that I would have to take daily for the rest of my life was an answer my doctor was all too willing to push as the solution to my problems. Between what I would have paid out of pocket and what my insurance would have covered, it would have added up to tens of thousands of dollars. Plus, I would have been tied to a prescription drug for the rest of my life, with all the possible side effects and health detriments.

When your doctor tells you something, of course, you're inclined to listen. But something about going on a cholesterol drug at age 17 seemed a bit off, and as it turns out, most medical schools across the country require absolutely no nutritional education![v] After a little research, I found there are other ways to reduce your cholesterol. One of the best: oatmeal. Every morning, for almost 15 years now, I have eaten oatmeal for breakfast. For variety, I mix it with different ingredients like shredded coconut, fruit, sunflower seeds, cacao nibs, peanut or almond butter, cinnamon, nutmeg.... It's amazingly delicious and takes just a few minutes. And, without cholesterol drugs, I've dropped more than 120 points in my cholesterol reading, saving myself both the potential side effects of prescription drugs, as well as the excessive cost.

How about a second example? I was recently selected as an "Alternative Transportation Hero" by the transportation department at the University of Hawaii, where I teach in the MBA program. I was chosen because I commute to work on a bicycle. When asked why I bike commute, I gave many answers (including that it's just more fun than driving, but also including the ease of parking, the lack of traffic in bike lanes, the fact that it helps me stay in shape...), but the answer that interested them the most, since I am a business school guy and they thought it was funny, was that I'd saved at least $50,000 in after-tax income by bike commuting (rather than commuting in my own car) over the last 15 years.

The secondary impacts from the kinds of practices we may call "green living ideas" are nothing but positive: from helping to solve major socioeconomic challenges that pervade many communities (like obesity and other public health epidemics), to curbing and ultimately reversing climate change, alleviating species extinction, and creating good green-collar jobs. There are a lot of upsides here! If we can all live a little healthier, a little greener, and save money on wasteful things like plastic, utility bills, and gasoline, we directly benefit.

So let's commence the good life, shall we? We'll start with energy savings you can easily implement around your house, then move on to health improvements in the second part of this book. This book is very image-driven by design. Pictures can be worth a thousand words, as they say, and we know that people may be more likely to understand and remember something when they see it illustrated. For those inclined to the written word, we summarize most of the green living ideas presented below, and of course provide links to supporting literature on the Internet wherever warranted. These shortened links, which may look like **bit.ly/74?*uLw,** will redirect you to the article. In the e-book version, click on them and open the article. In the print edition, you'll have to type them.

Symbols to know while reading this book:

SAVE

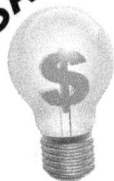

POTENTIAL ECO-SAVINGS: With this symbol, we'll outline the financial savings you may enjoy if you take on the habits and strategy being outlined. Sometimes, these are the financial savings over the life of the product that we're talking about. Sometimes, it's an estimated annual savings for an average family of four. Rates are based on Hawaiian Electric Company's energy costs at the time of this writing. Actual savings may vary. If you want to see how we made these calculations, refer to the Green Living Ideas summary links at the end of each chapter.

GO ONLINE: This symbol means you can refer to a link for additional information.

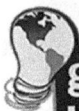

green living ideas

LEARN MORE: This symbol will give you an article covering the subject matter of that chapter in more detail, including calculations on cost savings.

SECTION I
Money-Saving
Green Living Ideas

CHAPTER 1
Your Refrigerator

Your refrigerator likely ranks in the top five energy users in your home. Follow these methods, and whatever fridge you own, it will use less energy, save you money, and still get the job done.

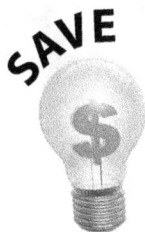

$492/year–$1,179/year

1 Practice the 2/3 full rule

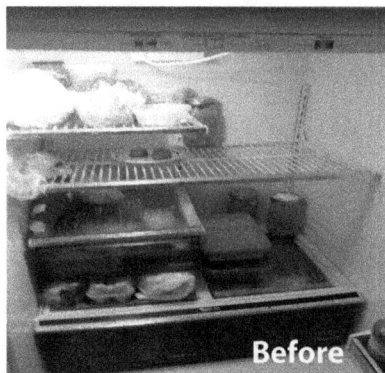

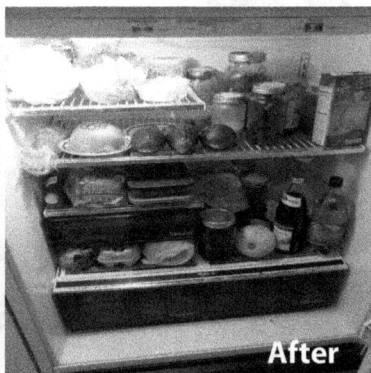

Before | After

By keeping the fridge and freezer at least 2/3 full, only 1/3 or less of that air can leak out. This is especially important if you and your family frequently open the doors.

2 Clean your condenser coils 2-3 times per year

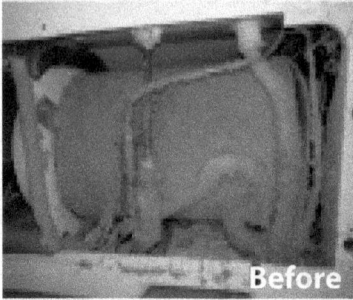

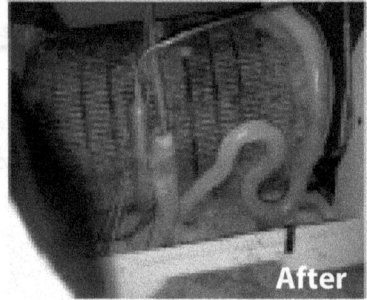

Before · After

Estimates are that you can save 15% of the electricity that the fridge uses if you keep the condenser coils clean, which could translate to an annual savings of $62 per year!

> To learn more about how to clean your condenser coils, visit: http://greenlivingideas.com/2014/07/22/clean-refrigerators-condenser-coils/

3 Make sure there's airflow around your fridge

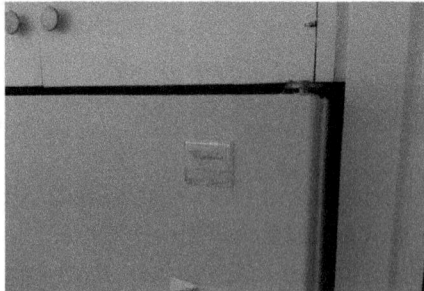

If you store a bunch of stuff on the top and sides of your fridge, it will keep your fridge working harder to get rid of the hot air created by the cooling process. So keep it clearer, and it will work more easily and use less electricity.

4 Keep an eye on frost buildup

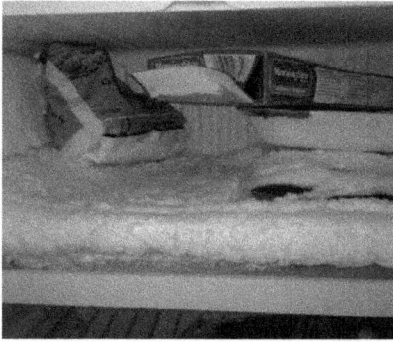

If the frost building up in your freezer is 1/4" or thicker, it's time to thaw and get rid of that frost — it's making your appliance work harder than it needs to.

5 Don't store open liquids — it causes frost buildup

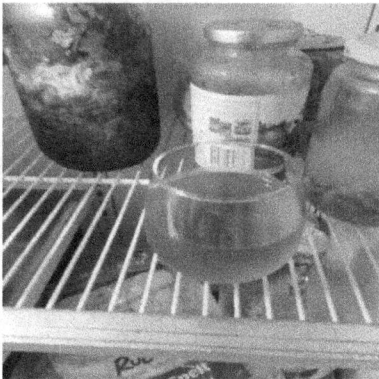

Avoid putting liquids in your refrigerator or freezer that don't have a lid. It will cause your appliance to work harder and could cause frost to build up, which in turn makes it work even harder and use even more energy. *So do yourself a favor and put a lid on it!*

6 Peek and grab

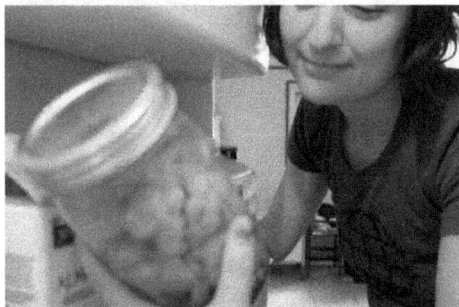

Roughly 7% of the energy used by your fridge can be attributed to the door simply being open and closed. So to help save energy and money, don't leave the fridge door open longer than it needs to be.

7 Strongly reconsider a second fridge

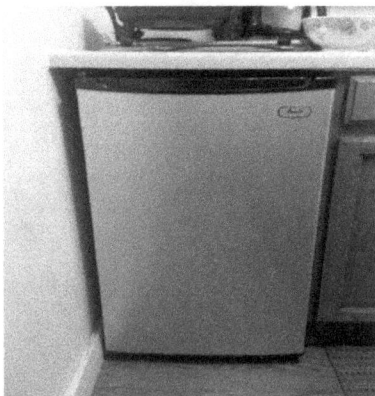

Even mini fridges can use upwards of 500 kWh of energy per year and cost you hundreds. If you have a second fridge for just a few things, strongly consider selling it and just using one fridge.

8 Skip the automatic icemaker

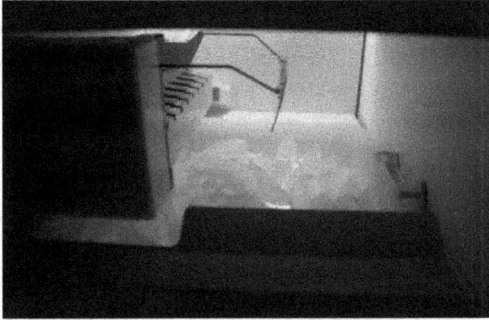

Automatic icemakers may cause your fridge/freezer to consume anywhere from 14%-20% more energy and could cost you as much as $437.31 per year! Our advice is to turn off your automatic icemaker and use ice trays instead.

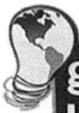

green living ideas To learn more about ways to make your refrigerator more energy efficient, visit GreenLivingIdeas.com/2014/09/25/ efficiency-tips-for-your-fridge-and-freezer/

CHAPTER 2
Food Storage

In this chapter, we'll show you ways you can save a lot of money and reduce your body's chemical burden by changing some of your food storage and handling habits.

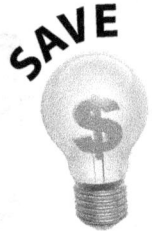

$2,200/year

1 Stop petrochemical additions to your food

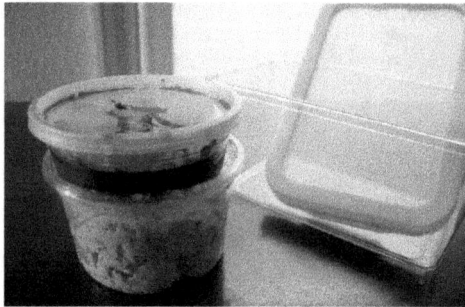

Plastic containers may be a cheap way to store your leftovers, but if you aren't careful they could be adding a petrochemical "seasoning" to your food. This is because some plastics will leach chemicals like BPA, antimony and phthalates which are not good to consume. So to be safe, skip the plastic entirely and use Pyrex, Mason jars, or other glass containers. If you use plastic, only use plastic Tupperware that is labeled with #5 or #7, so as long as the #7 is designated as BPA-free.

2 Be careful microwaving your leftovers

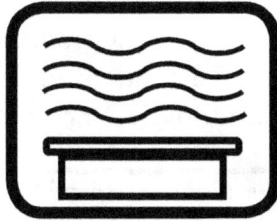

"Microwave-safe"? The jury is still out on this one, but when a plastic food storage item is marked as microwave safe, all it really means is that the plastic itself won't melt if you put it in the microwave. The designation of "microwave-safe" (pictured above) means NOTHING in terms of whether it will cause the plastic to leach chemicals into your food. Microwaving in Pyrex containers (as long as you don't put the lid in with it) is a better option than microwaving in plastic of any kind.

3 Save money by decreasing food waste

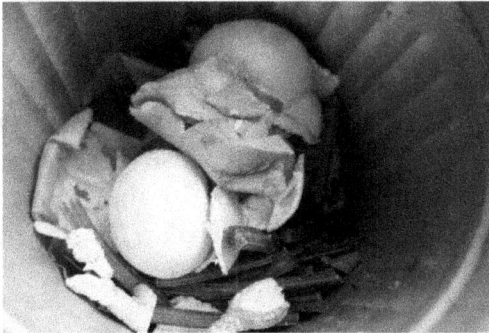

According to the Natural Resources Defense Council (NRDC) the average American family of four throws away anywhere from \$1,350-\$2,275 worth of food per year![vi] The first thing to know is that the "expiration date" printed on most packaged foods is not usually an actual expiration date:

it's usually more of a "best by" date. In other words, crackers may lose a bit of their crunch, but they're likely not truly "expired." Obviously, we can't tell you to eat expired food, but the science is definitely clear on this: most products remain good well past their "expiration date." For more information check out these two articles from EatDrinkBetter.com:

http://eatdrinkbetter.com/2011/12/28/reduce-food-waste-part-1/ and
http://eatdrinkbetter.com/2013/11/23/how-long-fridge-food-lasts-past-expiration-date/

4 Use smart food storage habits

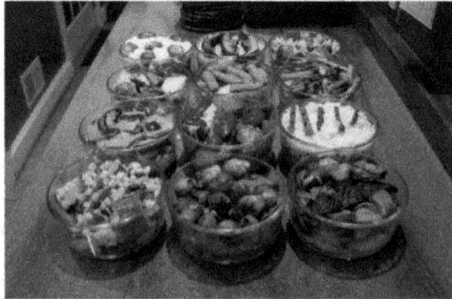

No matter what food you make, let it cool to room temperature before you put it in the fridge, otherwise, hot food placed in your fridge will make the fridge use more energy. If you are defrosting something, take it out of the freezer and put it in the fridge so that when it thaws out, it helps the fridge stay cold, saving energy.

5 Use reusable grocery bags/repurpose your plastics

Plastic, including the bags given out at grocery stores, is made from oil. While the plastic industry wants us to think

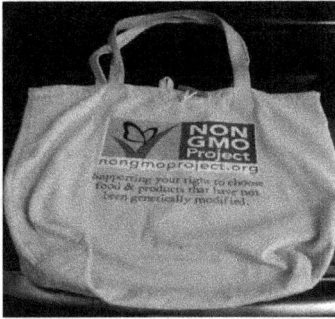

recycling is the answer to this waste, the truth is that a paltry 9% of plastics are actually recycled.[vii] The rest go out into the world, clogging sewer drains and waste management facility machinery, killing wildlife, contaminating and being a scenic blight in otherwise beautiful places. Our recommendation is to switch over to reusable grocery bags. In many places, stores give a 5 or 10 cent discount if you bring your own bag. In our house, that translates into more than $50 a year in savings.

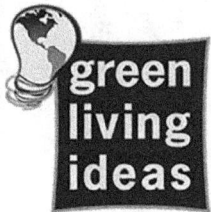

green living ideas If you'd like to learn more about how to save money by saving food, visit GreenLivingIdeas.com/2014/09/25/5-money-saving-sustainable-food-strategies/

CHAPTER 3
Efficient Cooking

You can save money on electricity when you cook by adopting a few easy habits. These will not only save you directly by making your cooking more efficient, they'll keep you from spending extra money on cooling your home, since you'll avoid using excess heating in the cooking process.

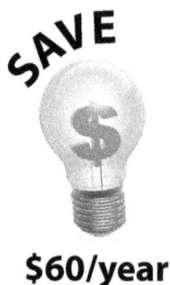

SAVE

$60/year

1 Match pot to burner size (don't cook the air!)

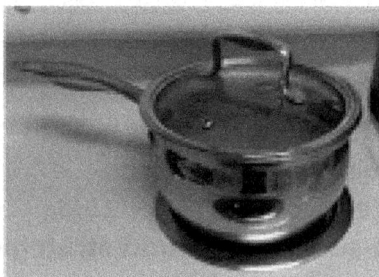

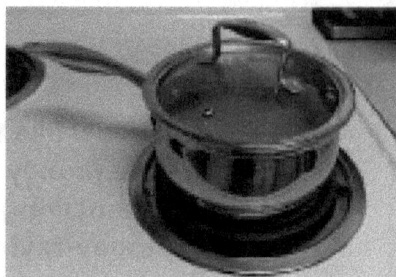

The difference is subtle, but note that the pot on the right doesn't touch all the coils—that's wasted energy, and money. If you cook a small pot on the large coil, you're wasting 30-40% of the electricity needed.

2 Use the right appliance

Comparison table of the energy costs of cooking the same meal by several methods

Appliance	Temperature	Time	Energy	Cost*
Electric oven	350°F	1 hr.	2.0 kWh	69¢
Convection oven	325°F	45 min.	1.39 kWh	48¢
Cooktop/ frying pan	420°F	1 hr.	0.9 kWh	31¢
Toaster oven	425°F	50 min.	0.95 kWh	33¢
Crockpot	200°F	7 hrs.	0.7 kWh	24¢
Microwave oven	"High"	15 min.	0.36 kWh	12¢

Cost assumes 34.5¢/kWh for electricity
(Adapted from ACEEE, Consumer Guide to Home Energy Savings, 1999)

3 Check your reflectors

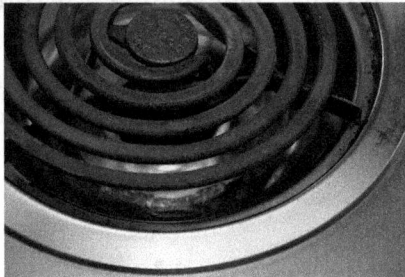

The metal drip trays underneath your stove burners serve two purposes. First, they catch spillover drips from your cooking. Secondly, they make your stove more energy efficient by reflecting heat back up to the pot or pan you're cooking in.

the point of having holes and rust, your stove won't use energy efficiently. Adding aluminum foil will help to make it as efficient as possible.

> Check out this article to learn more about adding aluminum foil to your stove's reflector drip pans: http://greenlivingideas. com/2014/05/13/adding-aluminum-foil-stoves-reflector-drip- pans/

4 Use your oven efficiently

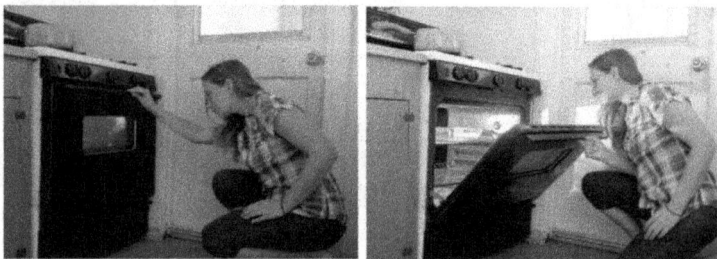

You can be more energy efficient by using the oven light to check your food creation (left, above). Opening the door causes the oven to work harder and use more energy to reheat itself (right, above). Every time you open the oven door, the internal temperature can drop 25-75 degrees and it will require more time to fully cook your food. We recommend that before cooking, test to make sure the oven light will show you what you need to see when cooking your food.

5 Capture residual heat

If you use the self-cleaning option, use it right after you bake something else. This way, you'll use the heat you have built up in the oven!

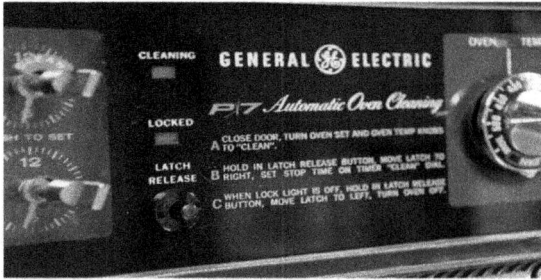

6 Consider cast iron

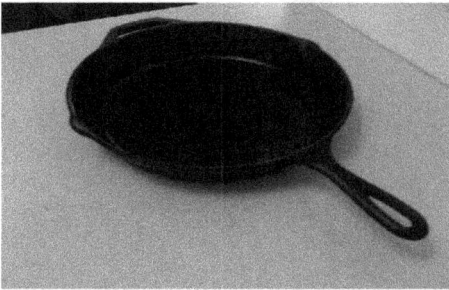

Cast iron cookware is a healthier option than many other types, and has some energy efficiency benefits. You can cook on a lower heat setting with cast iron than you can with nonstick or stainless steel cookware, and it won't scratch and flake material into your food like Teflon pans. When you scratch a Teflon pan it begins a slow, steady and inevitable process wherein Teflon chips off and enters your food while you cook with it. MMM...Teflon seasoning...zesty!

See "How Toxic is Teflon?" here: http://greenlivingideas. com/2012/06/13/how-toxic-is-teflon/

7 Pre-measure your water for boiling

If you make tea, use a French press for coffee, or boil specific amounts of water for a recipe, pre-measuring how much you need will save you both energy and money. This allows you to boil exactly the amount of water needed for your beverage and not a drop more. The perfect pour...every time.

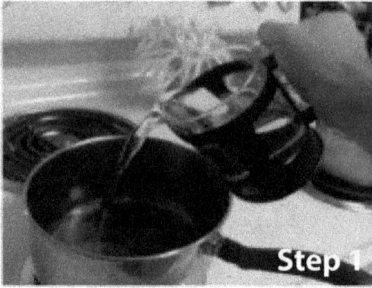

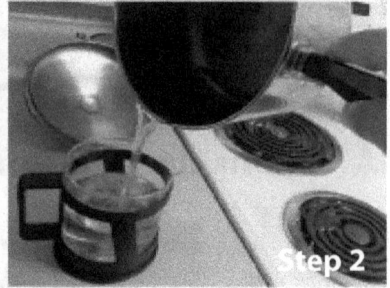

Step 1 Step 2

8 Or...cold brew coffee and tea

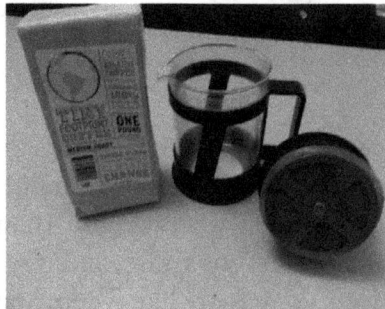

A great way to save money and still start your day with a cup of coffee or tea is to cold brew it. Just take a French press, fill it with water, put ground coffee or a tea bag in it, and let it brew on your counter overnight. When you wake up the next morning, your drink will be ready to go, saving you time and money!

For cold brew coffee ideas, see: http://feelgoodstyle.com/2014/06/24/diy-iced-coffee-cold-brew-joe-summer/

9 The pasta principle

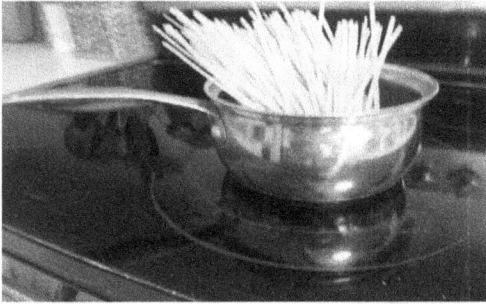

The next time you're cooking some pasta, rice, oatmeal, or other grain, use what we call the "pasta principle!" Turn off the burner after only cooking for a few minutes and put a lid on the pot. The grains will absorb the residual heat and soften up, and it should only take a few more minutes than if you were to leave the burner on the entire time you were boiling. Doing so will reduce the amount of energy used to prepare your meal and you will still get the same results. Brown rice and other dense grains may need more cooking time than pasta, but will likely cook just fine with the same strategy and a few extra minutes.

10 Cover foods while cooking

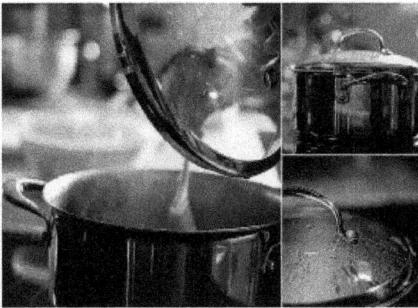

By covering your foods while you cook you will reduce the overall cook time and the amount of energy needed to cook it. Plus, you will prevent food from splashing onto your stove or countertops and save yourself from the added cleanup.

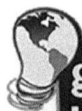

green living ideas

If you're looking for more ways to save money around your kitchen, visit GreenLivingIdeas.com/2014/09/27/tips-for-efficient-cooking/

CHAPTER 4
Washing Dishes Efficiently

Hot water is a triple whammy for your utility bills. First, it costs money to get the water (water bill). Second, it costs money to heat that water (electricity or gas bill). And last, it costs money to dispose of that water (sewer bill). Learning how to wash dishes more efficiently can save you thousands of dollars during your lifetime, and help significantly reduce your carbon and water footprints.

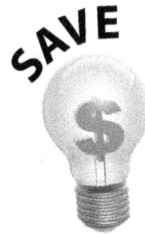

$71.51/year

1 Use your dishwasher efficiently

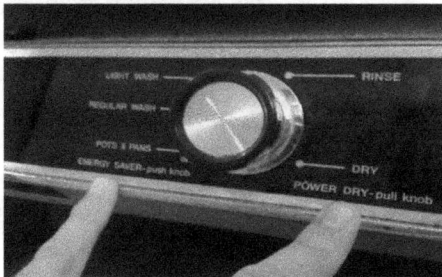

Using the proper dishwasher settings is one of the easiest and fastest ways to save both money and energy. Check your dishwasher and change the settings so that the heated dry option is turned off: dishes will dry just the same, just a little more slowly. If you want to help expedite the drying of your dishes, just open the dishwasher door when the dishwasher is done and leave it open a crack.

2 Practice good habits with your dishwasher

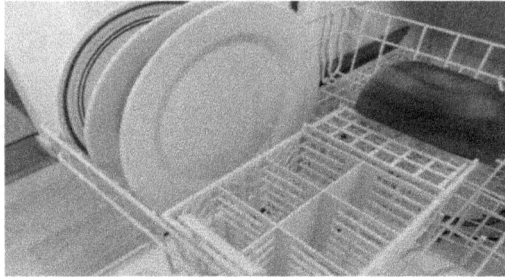

Scrape your dishes of excess food and other debris, but don't pre-wash them. It's unnecessary and wasteful. Plus, it's extra work! Stack dishes facing inward. Just about all dishwashers are designed so that the spraying water and soap comes from the middle (both top and bottom), so if dishes are facing outward, they will not be as effectively cleaned.

3 Only run when it's full

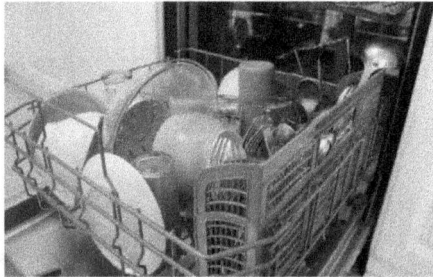

Your dishwasher will use the same amount of water and energy regardless of how full it is. So to use both as efficiently as possible, only run your dishwasher when it's full.

4 Hand washing? Follow grandma's strategies

Your grandmother had a little bin in her sink, right? Turns out, your grandma was quite the conservationist. The bin

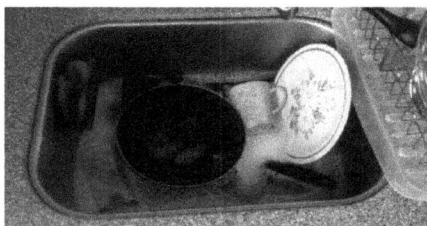

had soapy water and was for soaking her dirty dishes. Once they've been in there for a short while, they're remarkably easy to clean. You can take them out of there and quickly wipe clean with a soapy sponge before giving them a rinse or dipping them into the rinse bin. The amount of time you spend at the sink will be decreased, and the amount of heated water you use will be, as well. Savings all around!

5 Extend the life of your sponges

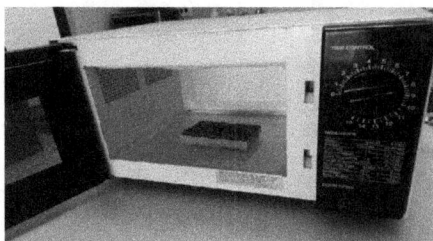

Sponges aren't exactly expensive, but over time, the money adds up. You can get more life out of your sponges by dampening them slightly and then microwaving them on high for 10 seconds or so. This also happens to be a terrific way to clean the caked-on splatters in your microwave — the steam escaping from that sponge will loosen food splatters and make the walls of your microwave a one-wipe cleaning job.

green living ideas If you're looking for more ways to save money around your kitchen, visit GreenLivingIdeas.com/2014/09/28/energy-saving-tips-for-washing-your-dishes/

CHAPTER 5

Greening Your Laundry

Doing laundry in an environmentally friendly way means you can save money and reduce your exposure to chemicals.

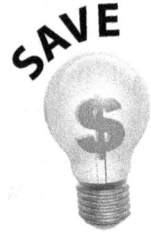

SAVE
$

$1,037/year

1 Wash and rinse in cold water

Water heater temperature set at 140°F			Water heater temperature set at 120°F		
Wash/rinse settings	kWh used	Average cost per load*	Wash/rinse settings	kWh used	Average cost per load*
Hot/Hot	8.3	$2.86	Hot/Hot	6.5	$2.24
Hot/Warm	6.3	$2.17	Hot/Warm	4.9	$1.69
Hot/Cold	4.3	$1.48	Hot/Cold	3.4	$1.17
Warm/Warm	4.3	$1.48	Warm/Warm	3.4	$1.17
Warm/Cold	2.3	$1.02	Warm/Cold	1.8	62¢
Cold/Cold	0.4	14¢	Cold/Cold	0.4	14¢

Cost assumes 34.5¢/kWh

Your parents may have washed everything in hot water, but that was before detergents were formulated to work in cold water. Now, just about all detergents, even if not labeled as Hot water also fades your clothes and therefore significantly shortens their useful life. Check out the chart on the previous page to see how much you're spending per load of laundry. The only reason you'd want to wash anything in hot water is if you have a lot of oil or grease on your clothes or if you have a serious stain and have pre-treated that stain with a stain remover. Otherwise wash cold. And ALWAYS rinse cold. Rinsing in anything else is a complete waste.

2 Wash full loads, not partials

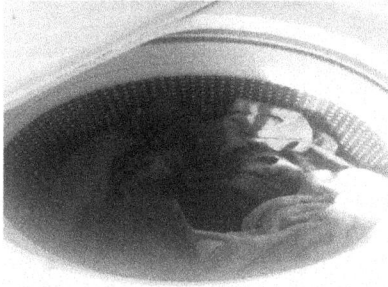

Did you know that your washing machine uses virtually the same amount of energy regardless of how full you fill it? To help reduce the amount of energy your home consumes, be sure to wash full loads instead of multiple smaller ones. You'll save not only energy and money, you'll save water as well. Cold water means no color running, so it is easier to do large loads.

3 Drying your clothes

Your clothes dryer is one of the biggest users of energy in your home, so to save money, try embracing a really awesome clean tech innovation: solar powered clothes dryers! That's right, we are referring to clotheslines (and in-house clothes drying racks, for folks who don't have the outdoor option). The average family switching to hanging clothes to dry can save more than $500 per year.

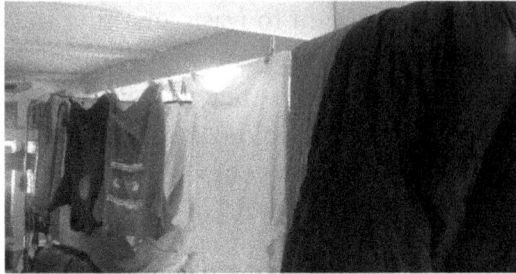

See http://greenlivingideas.com/2014/09/01/5-effective-tips-hanging-clothes-dry-inside/ for effective tips to line dry clothing indoors.

4 Set the dryer to the "auto dry" setting or dry for less time than you think you need

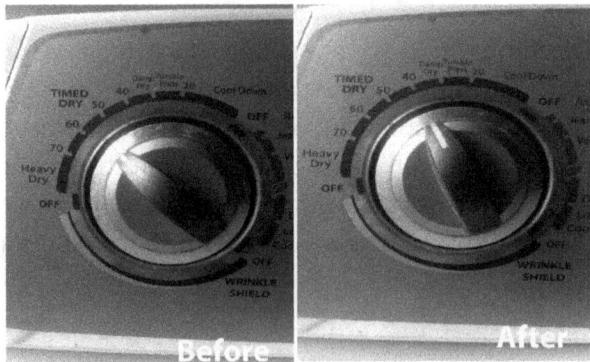

If your dryer has an auto-dry setting, use it. This will assure that when your clothes are dry, the dryer will turn itself off and not spend a bunch of extra electricity to continue to dry your already dry clothes. If you don't have an auto dry setting, set the dry time to less than you'd expect. Turn the buzzer on so you can check it when it's done. Turn it on for a few more minutes if needed.

5 Clean your lint screen between every load

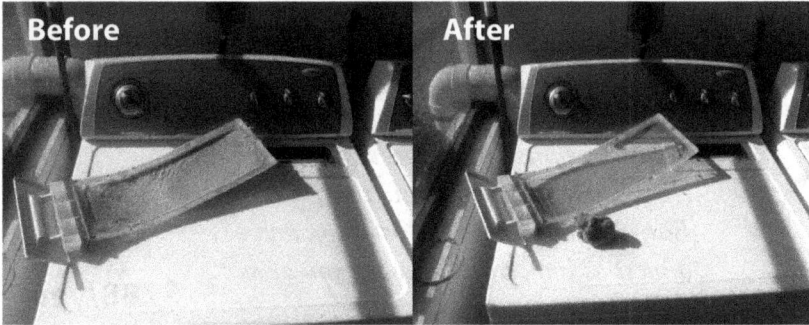

Before | After

Be sure to clean out the lint from your dryer's lint screen between uses. This will help to ensure good airflow and keep your dryer working efficiently. Clogged lint can be a fire hazard in your home, as well as a general health challenge for people sensitive to dust.

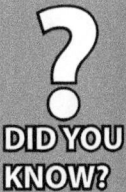

> **? DID YOU KNOW?**
> If you still really must use your dryer, you can save about 10% of the overall cost by making sure the lint screen, lint trap, and lint vent are cleaned out regularly. Check out this article from Green Living Ideas to see how easy it is: http://greenlivingideas.com/2014/08/14/clean-dryers-lint-trap-duct-screen

green living ideas **For more ways to green your laundry, visit GreenLivingIdeas.com/2014/09/23/ 3-easy-ways-to-green-your-laundry/**

CHAPTER 6
Going the Extra Mile

---

*Have a gas guzzler? You could save thousands of dollars and large amounts of carbon emissions by having a more eco-friendly car. You knew that, of course. But, did you know that **how** you drive is almost as important as **what** you drive?*

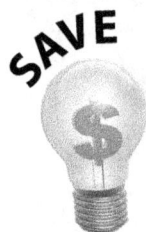

$ave

$288/year

1 Your tires

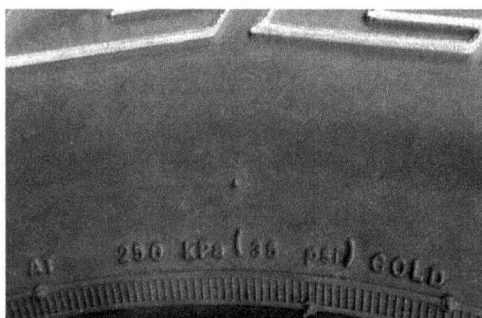

According to the U.S. Department of Energy (FuelEconomy. gov), your car's fuel efficiency will drop 0.3% for every PSI (pounds per square inch, a measure of pressure) each tire is underinflated (also, driving around on underinflated tires is unsafe).[viii] Your car tires will have a label on them for the recommended tire pressure, however, according to the U.S. Department of Energy, the proper inflation amounts are actually found in your owner's manual or the information on the inside of the driver door, so use these as your reference instead.

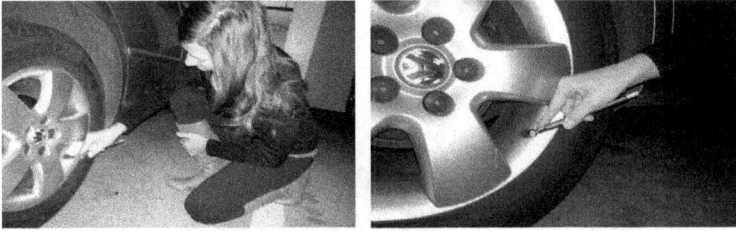

Testing your tire pressure is very easy. Many gas stations and every car mechanic will have a hose with a gauge attached with which you can check your pressure and fill your tires with air. Just unscrew the cap on your tire and apply the gauge to the valve. Hold in the gauge to pump air, and periodically release the gauge to check the pressure until you get it the right level.

2 Your engine

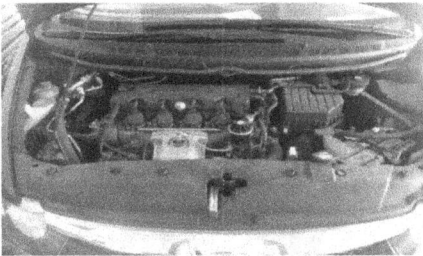

If your car is not properly tuned, it's like trying to exercise after eating fast food: not pretty. Proper maintenance of your car will help keep your car running efficiently. The DOE says that major maintenance problems, like a faulty oxygen sensor, can drop your fuel efficiency by as much as 40%. The best idea is for you to have your mechanic do a fairly regular comprehensive check to inspect for potential problems that might cause your fuel efficiency to drop. Regular maintenance is MUCH cheaper than all of that money you could lose by putting it off.

3 Slow down, Speedy Gonzales!

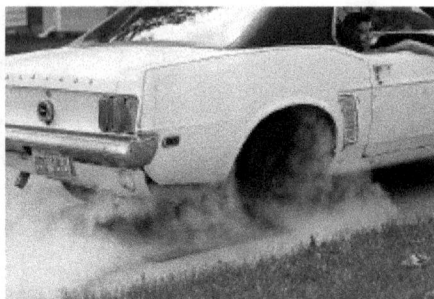

Love to drive aggressively? You're only costing yourself more in gas money. There is a concept called eco-driving (there are even driving schools specializing in it). The main tenets of eco-driving can more or less be boiled down to a few basics: accelerate gently, drive the speed limit, crack your windows if that's comfortable enough (instead of using A/C), lay off the gas and cruise if you see a red light ahead, and don't idle when parked.

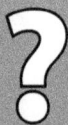

? DID YOU KNOW? Trade in a gas-guzzling SUV for a fuel-efficient car and you could save $20,000 over the next five years in fuel costs!

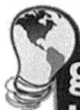

green living ideas For more ways to save money behind the wheel, visit GreenLivingIdeas. com/2014/10/09/going-extra-mile-eco-friendly-driving/

CHAPTER 7
Keeping Cool

Heating and cooling a home is typically one of the top three energy users contributing to high utility bills (alongside the fridge and the water heater). Use these strategies to reduce your heating and cooling costs.

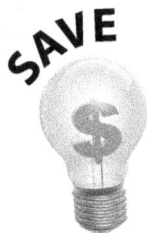

SAVE

$200/year

1 Keep heat-generating activities outside if possible

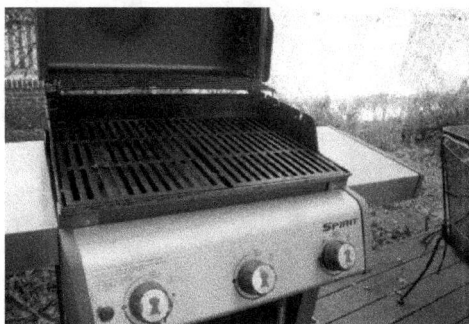

Activities like cooking and laundry will add ambient heat to your home, and thus cause your air conditioner to work harder, making that hot lunch a double whammy on your monthly electric bill.

2 Fans cool people, not rooms

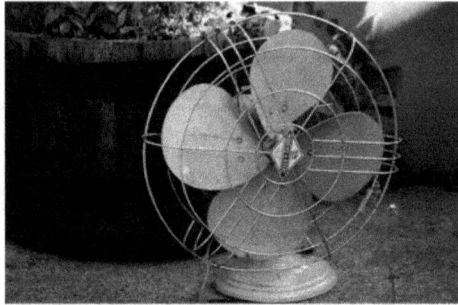

Fans are a great way to beat the heat, but they don't actually cool your room, they cool people by what is known as the "wind chill effect." As the breeze passes over your skin it causes moisture to evaporate, making you feel cooler. However, if you leave a fan on when people aren't in the room, you're actually making it hotter in there. So turn 'em off unless you are right there to enjoy them!

3 Keep heat away from your thermostat

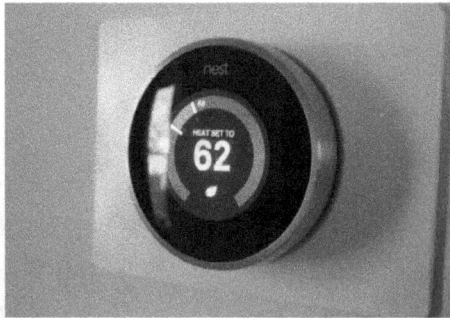

Your thermostat continually measures the temperature of the room relative to the temperature setting on the thermostat itself. If the room is warmer than the setting on the thermostat, your A/C kicks on to cool the room. However, if there are objects near the thermostat that give off heat (like electronics equipment) the thermostat may read a higher temperature than the room itself, which will cause your A/C to work harder, use more energy, and cost you more money.

4 Orient your blinds properly to deflect the sun

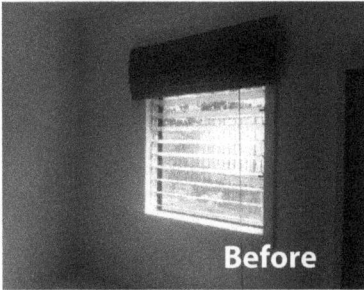

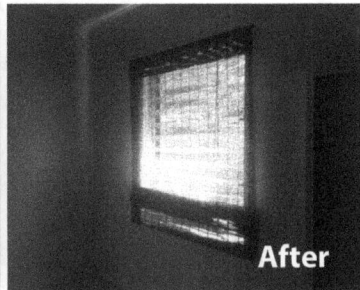

One of the best ways to keep your home cool on a hot day is to prevent the heat from the sun's rays from entering it in the first place. By properly orienting your blinds, you limit the amount of heat entering your home. While you're thinking about it, if you live in a hotter climate, maybe plant a shade tree outside the windows where you get the worst of the afternoon sun.

5 Be sure your windows and doors are properly sealed

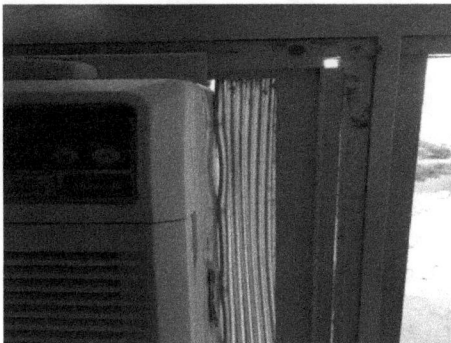

One of the best ways to ensure your home's A/C system is working efficiently is to check your doors and windows for drafts. Drafts in your home's doors and windows will allow warm outside air into your home while simultaneously allowing the cold air generated by your A/C system to escape. Check your seals on a regular basis to ensure that your system isn't working harder than it has to.

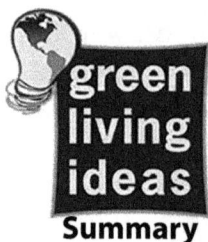

green living ideas
Summary

For more ways to beat the heat, visit GreenLivingIdeas.com/2014/10/09/5-energy-tips-beat-heat/

SECTION II
Green Living Ideas for Your Health

CHAPTER 8
The War on Germs

Germs are big business. Watch the ads on TV, with the scary, highly magnified images of creepy little bean-shaped bacteria with weird bumps on them and hairy appendages all around, and you may be tempted to a life of germaphobia.

Relax. Bacteria are EVERYWHERE, and no matter what you do, you'll never get them out of your house. Don't fret...here are some strategies to help reduce your chances of getting sick from bacteria, and to reduce your exposure to toxic stuff that marketers are selling you to kill those germs.

1 Your cutting board

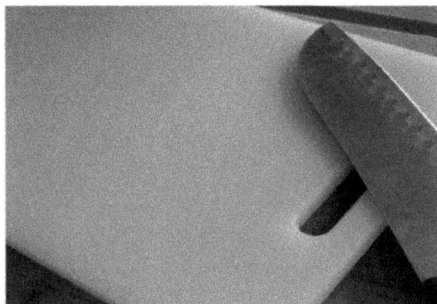

Your cutting board is a place where bacteria hide. If it has a lot of grooves crisscrossed into it, you may have a safe harbor for bacteria. When you clean that cutting board, the soap and scrubbing action you use may not get deep enough into those cuts, allowing bacteria to escape the cleaning process. Additionally, small chips of plastic may break off and get into your food. We recommend replacing any plastic cutting boards with bamboo cutting boards. Unlike plastic, bamboo has natural antibacterial properties. The grooves cut into a bamboo cutting board can be repaired with a little sprinkle of salt, or sand paper, and a little scrubbing to smooth out the grooves.

2 Your soup

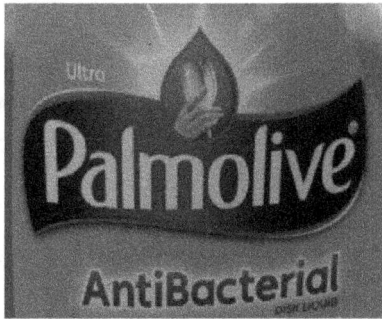

Both the American Medical Association and the American Academy for Microbiology say there is zero difference in the results of washing with regular soap compared to soaps with antibacterial ingredients. Plus, it's terrible for you! See the "Did You Know?" callout below.

> **DID YOU KNOW?**
>
> One of the main ingredients found in soaps labeled "anti-bacterial" is triclosan, which is classified by the Food and Drug Administration as a "probable carcinogen" (in laymen's terms, that means it probably causes cancer). It does nothing more than regular soap, so they're selling you a potentially cancer-causing chemical solely as a marketing ploy!

3 Your knife rack

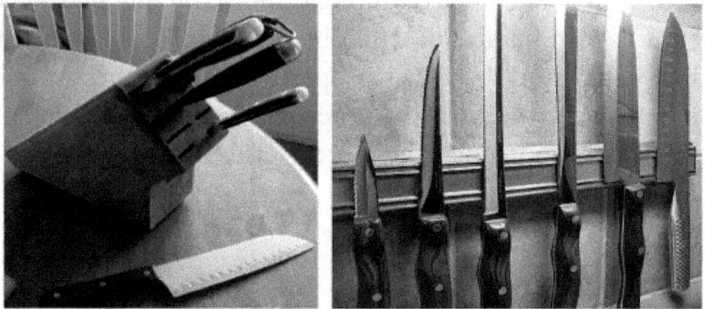

The knives you use for chopping vegetables and prepping ingredients are often a major source of bacteria, at just the wrong time — right before you eat. Knife blocks and similar ways of storing your knives can become bacterial havens: after all, it's virtually impossible to clean inside the slots of a knife block. We recommend storing your knives on a magnetic strip attached to your wall. The magnetic strip is easy to clean so your knives should be cleaner and safer to use as a result.

CHAPTER 9
Ingredients

Ever looked at the ingredient label on a box of cookies or a sports beverage? Ever wondered what FD&C Yellow #2 really is? The U.S. Food and Drug Administration has allowed a lot of questionable ingredients to become fully approved as additives for our food and personal care products. Here, we try to give you some guidelines about shopping and finding stuff that will be best for you and your family.

1 Your food

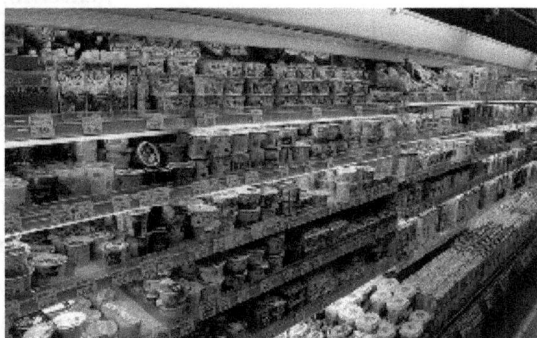

Can you pronounce it? If not, should you be eating it? Take a quick look at the ingredients on the first box or can of food you find in your pantry. You may find ingredients such as "enriched" wheat flour, glucose, high fructose corn syrup, xanthan gum, ascorbic acid, maltodextrin or something called "flavoring." When you buy packaged goods, try to find stuff that has ingredients you can pronounce and that you know, so you can avoid some of those chemicals.

2 Your personal care items

How many carcinogens are in your lipstick? Between the unknown effects of many additives and the lack of labeling requirements, the answer is: who the heck knows? Below, we do our best to identify the worst of the worst ingredients, broken down by personal care item.

Personal Care Item	Ingredient of Concern	Potential Health Effects
Soap	Triclosan	Probable carcinogen
	Triclocarban	Thyroid and endocrine disruption
	1-4 Dioxane	Probable carcinogen
	Bronopol	Thyroid disruption
Deodorant & Antiperspirant	Aluminum	Alzheimer's
	Fragrance	Who knows? "Fragrance" is a catchall term for more than 200 types of chemicals
Lip Balm	Retinyl Palmitate	Facilitates cancer cell growth when exposed to sun
	Retinol	Facilitates cancer cell growth when exposed to the sun

Personal Care Item	Ingredient of Concern	Potential Health Effects
	Vitamin A (synthesized)	Facilitates cancer cell growth when exposed to the sun
Sunscreen	Oxybenzone	Probable carcinogen
	Aerosol spray of any kind	Chemical inhalation hazard for yourself and others around
	Benzalkonium or Benzethonium Chloride	Endocrine and immune system disruption
	Retinyl Palmitate, Retinol, Vitamin A (synthesized)	See lip balm, above
Toothpaste	Triclosan	See soap, above
Shampoo	PEG, Ceteareth, or Polyethylene	Endocrine system disruption
	Parabens	Brain/nervous system. Also, probable carcinogen
	DMDM Hydantoin	Allergy and immunotoxicology
Dandruff Shampoo	Selenium Sulfide, coal tar, Ketoconazole, Salicylic acid	Known carcinogens
	Lead	Brain/nervous system damage

Personal Care Item	Ingredient of Concern	Potential Health Effects
	Phenacetin	Probable carcinogen
Hairspray	Nitromethane	Probable carcinogen
Cosmetics	Parabens	Brain and nervous system damage, carcinogenic
	SLS (Sodium Laureth Sulfate)	Opens pores to allow greater absorption of other chemicals
	DEA, as Cocamide or Lauramide	Becomes carcinogenic if mixed with nitrosating agents
	BHT, BHA	Banned in the EU
	Quaternium 15, TEA, MEA, Imidazolindinyl Urea	These form nitrosamines, so if mixed with DEA (above), it's a nasty combo!
Moisturizer	Benzalkonium or Benzethonium Chlorides	Endocrine and immune system disruption
	1, 4 Dioxane	Probable carcinogen
	Petrolatum	Banned in the EU
	Bronopol	Endocrine and immune system disruption

Personal Care Item	Ingredient of Concern	Potential Health Effects
Nail Care	Formaldehyde, Formalin, Toluene	Possible carcinogens
Anti-Aging Products	Bronopol, SLS, Propylene Glycol, Alpha and Beta Hydroxy Acids, Glycolic Acid	Endocrine and immune system disruption, among others
Diaper Cream	BHA, Sodium Borate, DMDM Hydantoin, Fragrance, Bronopol	All sorts of bad outcomes!
Acne Treatments	Parabens, Triclosan	Probable carcinogens
	PEG, Ceteareth, Polyethylene	Endocrine system disruption
Perfume	"Fragrance"	Who knows? See deodorants, above
	Diethyl Phthalate, Oxybenzone	Probable carcinogens
Aftershave	Oxybenzone	Probable carcinogen
	PEG, Ceteareth, Polyethylene, Parabens	Probable carcinogen
Shaving Cream	Triclosan	Probable carcinogen
	DMD Hydantoin, PEG, Ceteareth, Polyethylene	Allergy and other symptoms

Personal Care Item	Ingredient of Concern	Potential Health Effects
Dental Floss	PTFE, PFC	Bioaccumulate, likely human carcinogens
Painkillers	Parabens	Brain and nervous system, probable carcinogen
	Sodium Lauryl/ Laureth Sulfate	Allows greater absorption of other chemicals
	PEGs, artificial colors	Endocrine system disruption

Freaked out yet?

Our advice is not to go crazy. We like you sane and happy. But if you can reduce most of the chemicals you're exposed to here, your body will love you for it.

3 Fragrance

Household cleaning products may be full of chemical ingredients that manufacturers are not required to disclose. A manufacturer can list "fragrance" as an ingredient on a product when realistically, it could be one or 500 or 1,000 different chemical compounds blended together. The official reasoning is that it's a trade secret, but cleansers do not need any fragrance to be effective, and therefore we reject the notion that manufacturers should be able to list it instead of actually disclosing any of the 500 or so chemicals that it might actually be.

Lest you think I overstate the case, just consider this: The dishwashing cleanser sold under COSTCO's brand, Kirkland Signature, has a disclosure on its label (huge kudos to COSTCO for this transparency) that sends people interested in knowing about "fragrance" to this page: **http://bit.ly/165LLcw.** What you'll see there, is the list, as of 2015, of the 3,059 possible chemical ingredients used in "fragrance" during that year by manufacturers sold in the U.S. See Tip 1 in the Indoor Air Quality chapter for the brands we recommend.

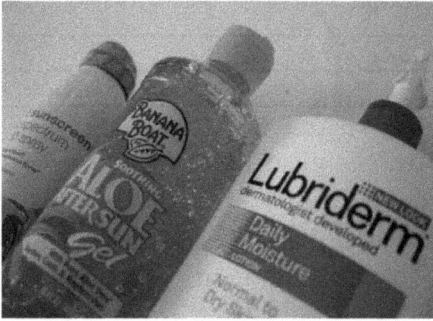

Check out page 67 of this book for recipes for DIY natural personal care and cleaning products you can make yourself!

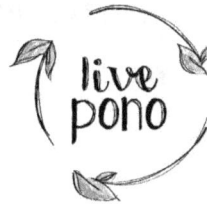

live
pono

You can also make a lot of your own cleansers. It's easier than you may think, and you can be sure of the ingredients (and save yourself a lot of money). Go to http://green livingideas.com/2008/04/27/natural-cleaning-recipes/

4 GMOs

Genetically engineered crops (also called genetically modified organisms, or GMOs) are crops that have been altered on a genetic (DNA) level for a variety of reasons, most commonly to withstand high doses of chemical herbicides and pesticides. Fields can then be sprayed with

GMO Ingredient	Commonly used for...
Corn or Soy Derivatives (unless labeled as organic)	
Maltodextrin	Thickening foods
Xanthan Gum	Bonding and thickening foods
Citric Acid	Flavoring and as a preservative, especially in soda
Monosodium Glutamate	Flavor enhancer
Lecithin (emulsifier usually derived from soy)	Stabilizing processed foods
Beta-Carotene (synthesized)	
Aspartame	Artificial sweeteners

Given the extra chemical residues that might come with GMO ingredients, and the controversy surrounding their use in our food and personal care products, you may just want to try to avoid using them.

5 Pesticides and Chemical Fertilizers

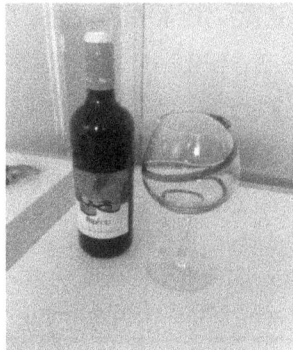

Organically grown foods are grown without using petrochemical pesticides, fungicides, herbicides, and fertilizers. Anything not labeled as organic was very likely grown with these chemicals, and the residue of those chemicals may make it into your food. Take wine, for example. Grapes are some of the most heavily sprayed crops in the world, so it's no real surprise that there will be residues of agricultural chemicals.

But if I were to tell you that the average number of pesticides that had detectable residues in wines found at a grocery store was 4, you might be perturbed, and never drink wine again. One wine tested even had 10 different pesticides in it.[ix] So what's a concerned oenophile (wine lover) to do? Look for the organic label.

Look, I'm organic!

CHAPTER 10
Your Indoor Air Quality

The air in our homes is often far more polluted than the air outside, where cars and buses are whizzing by. How is that possible? And how can you make it better?

1 Your cleansers

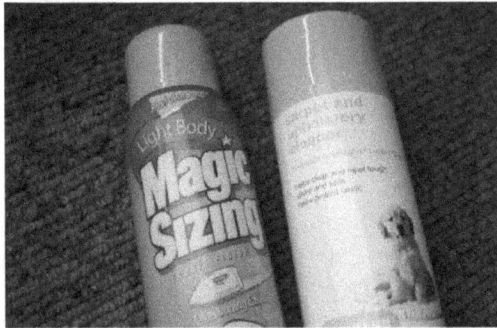

As we mentioned earlier, most cleansers can have a toxic brew of petrochemical ingredients, but did you know that skin exposure is only one of the many ways they can invade your body? If you've ever cleaned a small, windowless bathroom with a chlorine-based cleanser, you may have experienced fatigue, a headache, achy muscles, blurred vision, or any number of other symptoms. All of these and more may be associated with inhaling the fumes from your cleanser. The best piece of advice we can give is to let your local health food store act as a kind of filter for you and your family. Buy all your cleansers there, and you're more than likely to find the greenest, healthiest products around. Natural cleansers like vinegar and baking soda can clean bathrooms, kitchens, carpets, drains, and more.

Brands we trust:
- Bon Ami (they make a scrubbing powder that is a better alternative to Comet)
- Seventh Generation
- Method
- Dr. Bronner's

2 Your candles

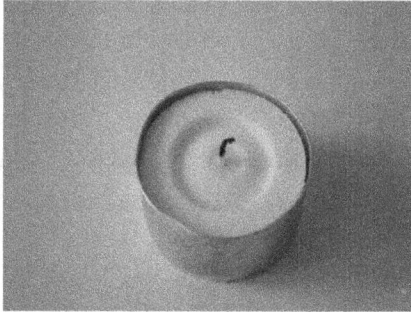

Did you know that breathing the aromatic and relaxing fragrance of a candle while you're taking a bath can be worse for you than breathing secondhand cigarette smoke. As it turns out, candles are pretty much as toxic as it gets, but since they're not food, their ingredients don't need to be placed on their labels in many places. Many candles, especially those made in China and imported, even have lead in their wicks. There is a reason leaded gasoline was banned in the United States — burning lead is terrible for our health! Look for candles that are 100% beeswax (organic if possible) as the only ingredient (if it doesn't say 100% beeswax, it may be

1% beeswax and 99% petrochemical paraffin). Also look for candles that have an organic cotton wick. It's the only way to assure that your exposure to breathing the gases of petrochemicals and heavy metals is as low as possible.

3 Your drains

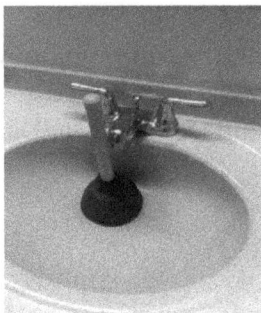

A clogged drain or sink is never convenient, but unclogging it doesn't have to be a difficult, chemical-ridden task. We recommend using a sink plunger to unclog your drains. They're inexpensive ($3-$10) and can be used on clogs for many years without using any chemical products.

> **See a cool video on how to most effectively use these here:** http://greenlivingideas.com/2014/05/15/unclog-drain-using-sink-plunger/

4 Your bedding

There's this phenomenon called "off-gassing." It's what you smell when you paint a new room. The problem? That smell is a nasty chemical that is turning from liquid additive to a gaseous and breathable form in your indoor air. Off-gassing is a big problem. Formaldehydes used in manufacturing furniture may continue to off-gas into your indoor air for many years, but the same phenomenon occurs with your bedding, where we spend roughly 1/3 of our lives. Our advice? Go organic. You may not be able to afford an organic mattress just yet, but at the very least, get yourself an organic pillow and organic pillowcases. They're affordable, readily available at many stores and online, and represent a great way to reduce your overall consumption of off-gassed chemicals.

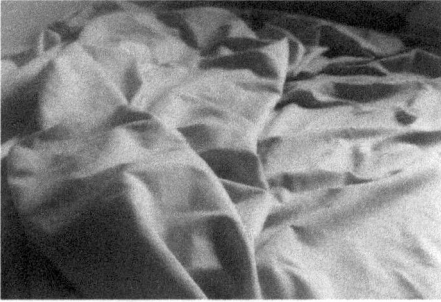

5 Dust

The dust in your house likely contains fairly high levels of PFOs (nonstick products like Scotchgard) and PBDEs (flame retardants). How does it get there? It's similar to off-gassing, but basically the chemicals in your house that are applied for one purpose (like flame retardants) do what chemicals do: they react with other things. As it becomes airborne, it may cling to other particles and rain down as dust. To keep levels of airborne chemicals in dust down in your house, just wipe down your hard surfaces every week with a damp cloth. Super easy, and super effective.

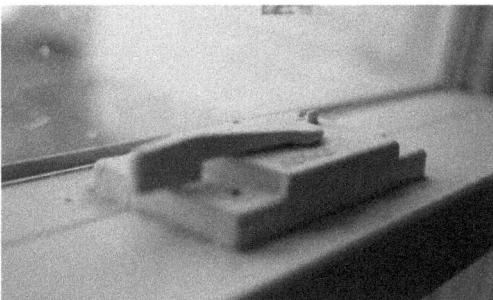

SECTION III
Additional Green Resources

CHAPTER 11
Additional Green Resources

This section has resources for additional financial savings you can find in your home that just didn't quite fit into the rest of the book.

1 Vampire power

Vampires on TV suck blood. In your house, however, your TV is very likely acting like a vampire, sucking energy right from the wall, even when it's off! The same is true for many other appliances that are not "on." The best way to tell for sure is to plug your appliances into a watt meter. But, for good measure, here's a handy guide on the next page, courtesy of Hawaiian Electric Company, on what some of your appliances may be costing you, just by leaving them off but plugged in. To avoid vampire power, consider getting power strips for your electronics, and turning them all off when not in use by turning the power strip button to the off position. This will stop your electronics from sucking electricity out of your wall and money out of your wallet.

Don't feel like the extra effort? A "smart strip" is different than a power strip, in that it has outlets that can stay on all the time, and other ones that turn off automatically when one control device is powered down. In other words, you can keep your clock turned on (the "hot" outlet), but when you shut your computer down (the "control" outlet), the smart strip will automatically cut off power to your speakers or printer or Xbox (on the "switched" outlets).

	POWER ON			STANDBY		
Description	Watts Used While "On"	Hours "On" Per Day	Cost Per Month*	Watts Used While On "Standby"	Hours on "Standby" Per Day	Cost Per Month*
32" LCD flat panel High Definition TV	143	7	$10.36	1	17	18¢
42" plasma High Definition TV	272	7	$19.71	1.4	17	25¢
34" tube TV	115	7	$8.33	4	17	70¢
DVD player	13	6	81¢	2.3	18	43¢
CD player	20	6	$1.23	3.1	18	58¢
Receiver	6.7	6	42¢	1.8	18	34¢
Power speaker	5.8	6	36¢	4.6	18	87¢
Mini stereo system	23	2	48¢	7	22	$1.59
Computer	75	5	$3.88	4	19	79¢
Computer printer— color ink jet	25	6	$1.52	5.25	18	98¢
Phone/ fax/copier combo	22	1	23¢	4.7	23	$1.12
Cordless phone	3	3	9¢	2.7	21	59¢
Cable box	16	6	99¢	15	18	$2.79
Microwave oven	1500	0.23	$3.88	3	23.75	74¢

*Cost assumes 34.5¢/kWh

2 Your computer

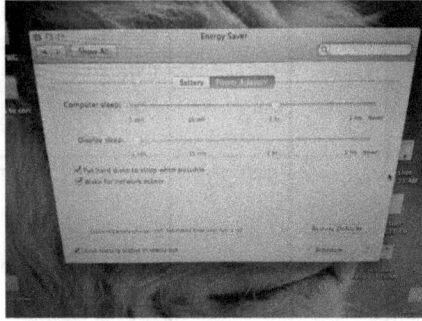

Did you know that by simply making sure that your computer goes into sleep mode after you're done using it you can save upwards of 423kWh per year? That's not the only thing you can do to make your computer more efficient. Be sure to avoid using your energy-wasting screen saver that doesn't even save your screen and turn down the brightness on your monitor. With these three easy tweaks you could save as much as $312 per year!

3 Dry cleaning

Ever walk into a dry cleaner and go, "What on earth is that smell?" The answer is perchloroethylene, or PERC, for short. It's a noxious gas that is used across the world for dry cleaning. As we have mentioned elsewhere, your nose is a pretty good guide to the toxins you're exposed to. The good news is you can avoid PERC. Wet cleaning is a growing eco-friendly and healthy alternative to traditional dry cleaning, and gets the same job done. Google "wet cleaning" in your area to see if any cleaners are offering this option, and use it preferentially over dry cleaning in order to avoid PERC. In addition, when shopping for clothes, read the labels and, for your own financial situation if nothing else, try to avoid clothing that can't be cleaned easily in a washing machine.

Many dry cleaning items can also be handwashed.

> **Check out more reading on PERC here:**
> http://bit.ly/oETB0M

4 Eating healthy on a budget

The main reason people give for not eating well is that it costs more. Sometimes that is true, as in the case of organic bell peppers: man, those are pricy! But, sometimes, you can eat really well and save money at the same time. Start by shopping at farmers' markets for good prices on local and organic produce. To save even more, you can ask vendors for imperfect goods: bruised tomatoes, or bananas with spots on them. Since they don't look perfect, oftentimes the vendor is unable or unwilling to put them out for sale, and would be more than willing to sell them to you for less than the perfect-looking stuff. The next strategy is to get to know the bulk bins at your local health food store. It's often much cheaper than packaged goods, plus it saves all that packaging waste. Finally, eat a more vegetarian diet. Beans and rice are healthy, delicious and very inexpensive staples. There are so many ways to save money. Check out the link below for more ideas.

> **Check out this article for some ways to do it:**
> http://bit.ly/17ZkbSZ

5 Saving money, washing hands

It is easy to overlook the washing of one's hands as a potential energy saver. After all, it's just a few seconds of

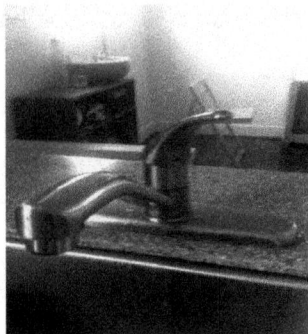

water, realistically, that you'll use. But this one habit can save you hundreds of dollars over the course of your lifetime. If you routinely turn on the hot water knob to wash your hands, odds are, the time it takes for that water to go through the pipes is long enough that the hot water won't even reach your hands. Instead, the hot water will just go to waste, coming from your water heater and running through potentially hundreds of feet of pipe but never ultimately getting to your hands. The heat will simply dissipate (and be wasted). So...get in the habit of turning on the cold water knob when washing hands. Simple!

SECTION IV

DIY Natural
Product Recipes

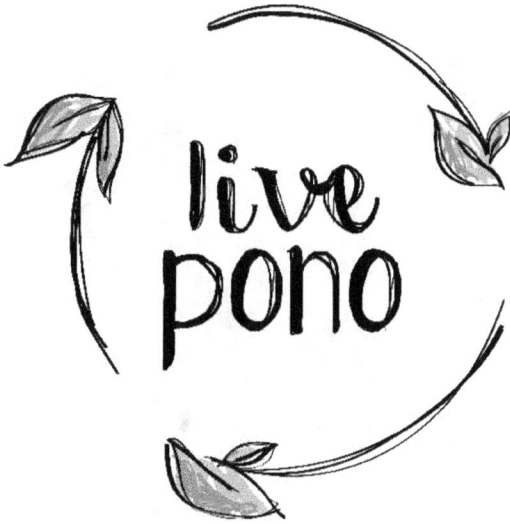

live
pono

Mouth Wash

2 cups filtered or distilled water or food-grade
hydrogen peroxide
10 drops essential oils (peppermint suggested)
Glass bottle or jar with secure lid

Directions:
1. Add essential oils to glass jar first, then water.

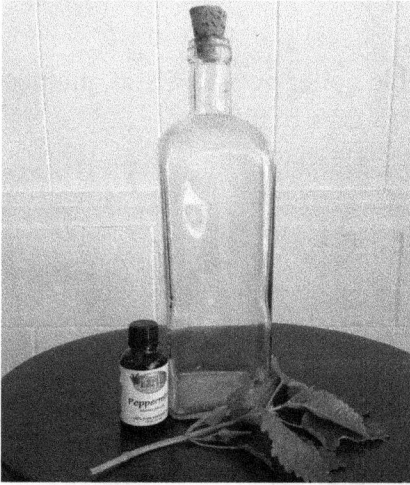

2. Shake before use. Keep lid closed lightly.

Luxurious Body Butter

Replenish and rehydrate your skin from head to toe! A little bit of this body butter goes a long way.

1/4 cup coconut oil
1/3 cup shea butter
1 tbsp. almond oil
10-20 drops essential oil of preference

Directions:
1. In a double boiler over low heat, melt coconut oil together with shea butter.

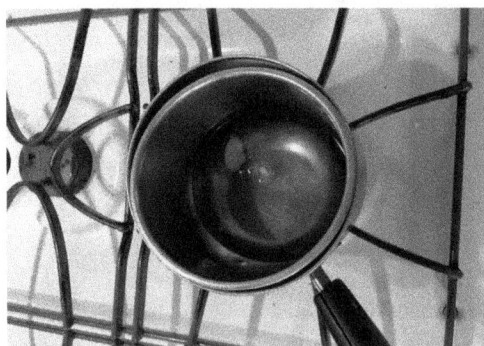

2. When fully melted, remove from heat and add almond oil and essential oils. Stir well and pour into a glass container.

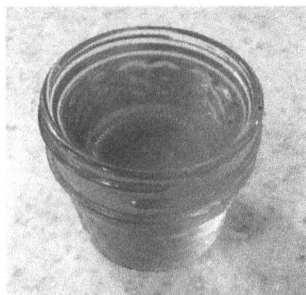

3. Put in the fridge one day to set up, stirring once or twice until mixture solidifies. Store in a cool place with an airtight lid on.

Suggested essential oils: Lavender and chamomile for relaxation and skin repair, rose and jasmine for a romantic scent, cedar wood or sandalwood for an earthy, woodsy scent, or clary sage for women's health and hormone balance.

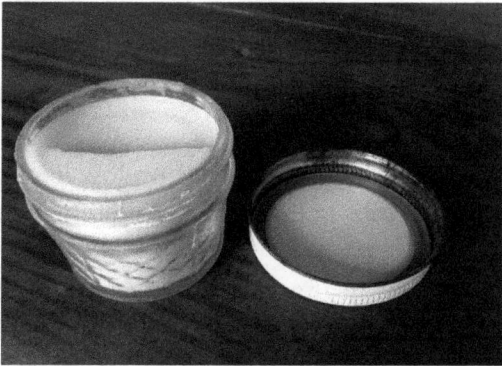

Peppermint Lip Balm

Hydrate your lips with simple, natural ingredients. This lip balm will harden into a similar consistency as your normal chapstick. You can make it softer by adding more oil, or harder by adding more wx.

1/4 cup almond oil
1 1/2 tsp. pure beeswax
1 tsp. vegetable glycerin
1-2 drops peppermint oil

Directions:
1. Combine the oil and beeswax on low heat in a double boiler until beeswax is completely melted.

2. Remove from heat and stir in glycerin. Blend with a whisk until creamy.

3. Add the peppermint oil and stir well to combine.

4. Pour quickly into small containers.

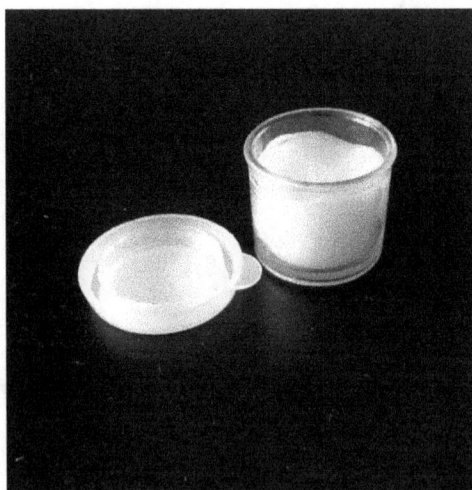

Coffee Coconut Body Scrub

1 cup coffee grinds (if using once-used coffee grinds, make sure to dry them out on a cookie sheet or paper towel to prolong the life of your scrub)
½ cup coconut oil, melted and cooled
¼ cup sugar

Directions:
1. Mix all ingredients. Store in an airtight and water-tight container.

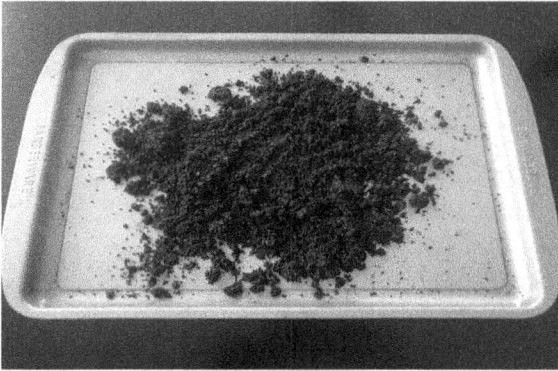

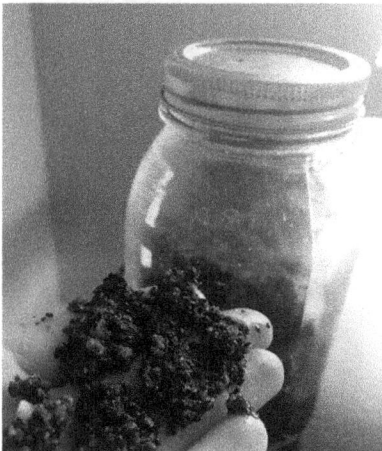

Laundry Soap

1 bar shredded castile soap
1 cup washing soda
1 cup borax
5 gallons water (for liquid soap)

Directions:
1. Grate bar of soap with a cheese grater.

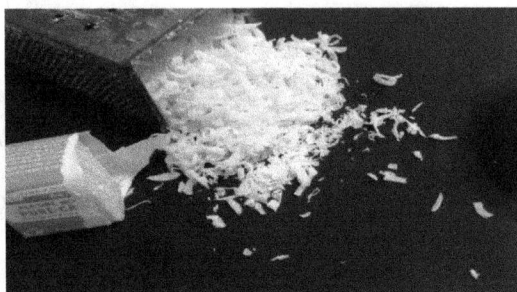

2. If making powdered soap (for warm/cold wash), mix washing soda and borax with shredded soap. Use about ¼ C for laundry.

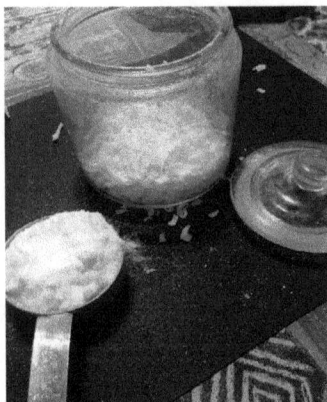

3. If making liquid soap (for cold/cold wash), boil 1 quart water in a pot and add shredded soap. Stir until soap dissolves. Add another quart of water to dissolved soap mixture.

4. Put 2 gallons hot tap water in a 5 gallon bucket. dissolve borax and washing soda into this hot water, then add the liquid soap mixture to the bucket. Add another 2 ½ gallons of water to make 5 gallons total, stirring well.

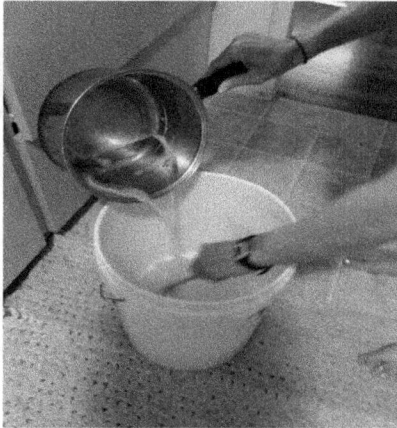

5. Transfer to jugs and use 1 cup for full load of laundry, ½ cup for HE washers.

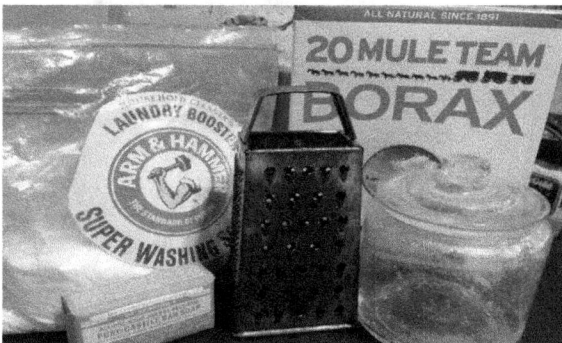

Lemon Salt Face Scrub

1 lemon
5 tbsp. sea salt
1 tbsp. olive oil

Directions:
1. In a small bowl, coat salt with olive oil (this prevents salt from dissolving).

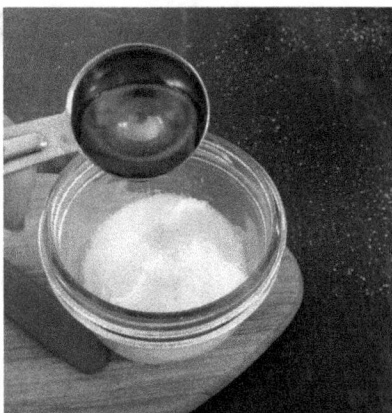

2. Cut the lemon in half and squeeze, mixing juice with salt and oil.

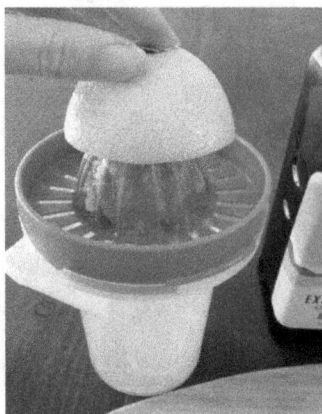

3. Store in a glass or plastic container. For best results avoid metal lids.

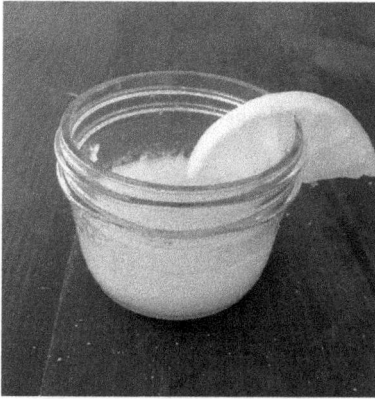

Shaving Cream

1/3 cups coconut oil
1/3 cups shea butter
2 tbsp. almond or olive oil
3 tbsp. liquid castile soap
2 tsp. baking soda
10 drops essential oils

Directions:
1. On low heat in a double boiler, melt coconut oil and shea butter.

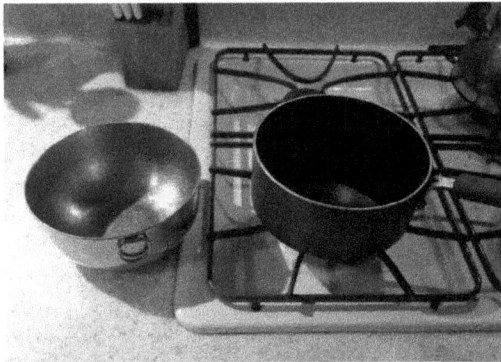

2. Remove from heat and add almond or olive oil.

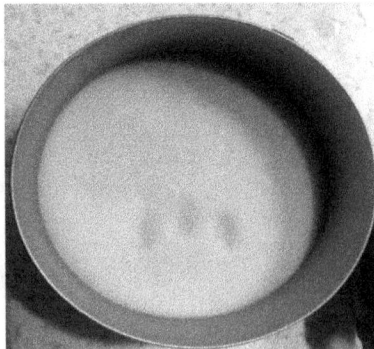

3. Transfer to a bowl and refrigerate until mixture is firm. This may take several hours.

4. When hardened, remove and mix with an electric beater. Start on low speed, and gradually increase gradually to high speed.

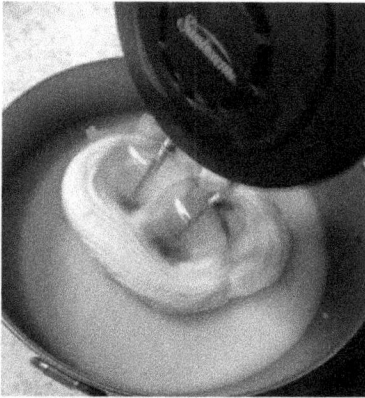

5. While mixing, add castile soap, baking soda, and essential oils.

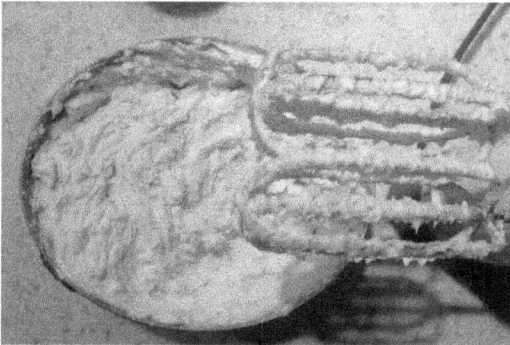

Cleaning Solution

4 cups vinegar
1/2 cup baking soda
2 squirts lemon juice
2 squirts dish liquid
4 cups water
Essential oils as desired

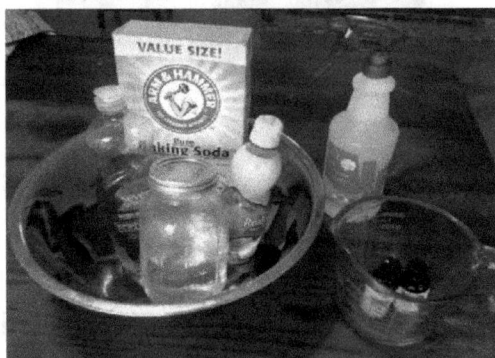

Directions:
1. Mix vinegar and baking soda in a LARGE bowl.

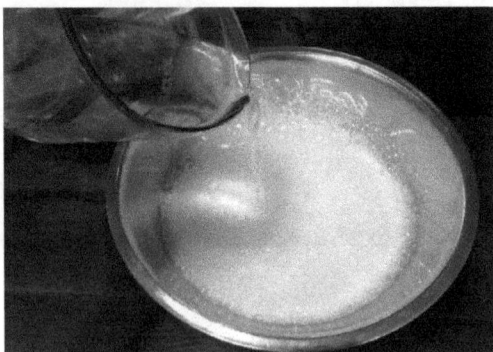

2. When foam dies, add other ingredients and mix well.

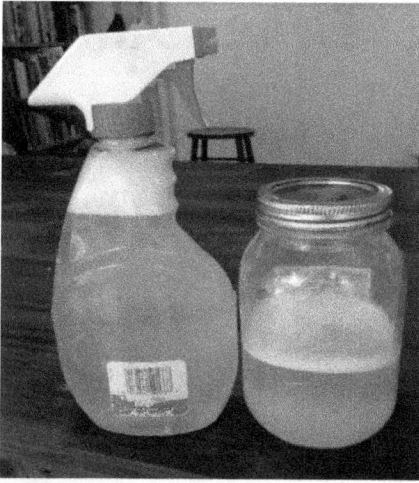

3. Put into a spray bottle. Use on all surfaces EXCEPT glass (it can cause streaks), granite, marble, and sealed concrete (it can dull the surface fairly quickly).

Dryer Balls

This is a reusable product to replace chemical–laden dryer sheets. Throw these balls into your dryer with your laundry to speed drying, fluff clothes, and take away static. Add a few drops of essential oils to the dryer balls before each use if you miss the scent of dryer sheets!

1 skein of wool yarn
Old panty hose
3-4 drops essential oils

Directions:
1. From yarn skein, make 3 small balls of yarn and secure the ends well.

2. Put the balls into the leg of old panty hose, separating each ball with a tight knot. WASH IN HOT WATER AND DRY.

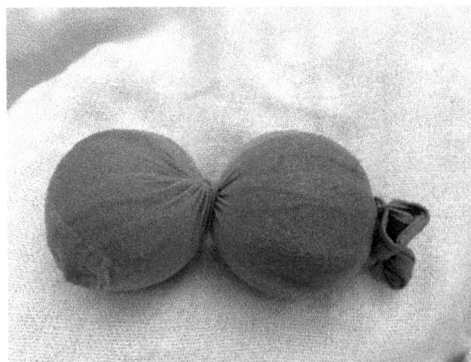

3. After washing and drying, remove balls from the panty hose. They should have a felted appearance.

4. Put a few drops of essential oil on them and throw them into your dryer with your laundry to speed drying, reduce wrinkles, reduce static, and add natural fluff and scent.

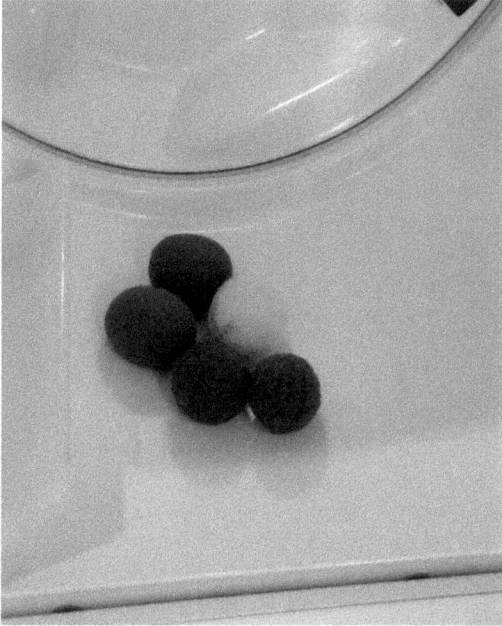

Pono Product Guide

If you prefer to buy your products, here's a quick reference guide to the personal care products we recommend.

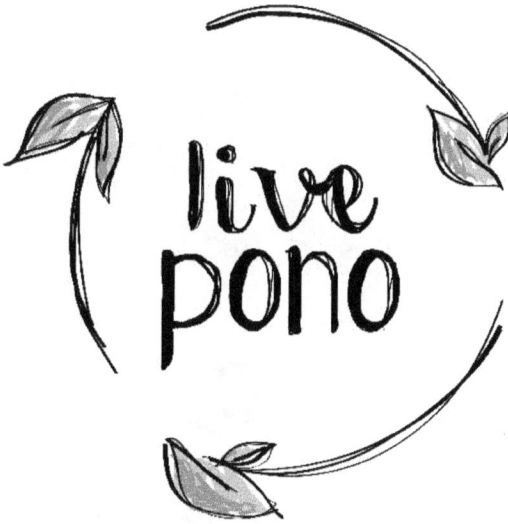

Lip Balm

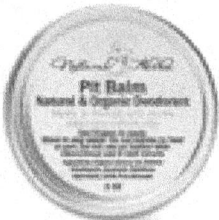

Ingredients to avoid:
Retinyl palmitate, retinol, and synthetic Vitamin A

Pono choice:
Badger Cocoa Butter Lip Balm

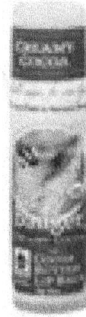

Why we love it:
Organic and Fair Trade (30% Fair Trade), the ingredients are great, and the larger size (0.25 oz. vs. 0.15 oz. for most other lip balms) means more product, less plastic, and more bang for your buck.

Deodorant

Ingredients to avoid:
Aluminum, fragrance

Pono choice:
Natural Aloha Pit Balm

Why we love it:
Great ingredients, made locally (with aloha!) and a plastic-free tin make this deodorant our top choice.

Runner-up (especially if using your hand to apply deodorant doesn't appeal to you: EO. Organic ingredients, yummy essential oils, at a very reasonable price point.

Shampoo and Conditioner

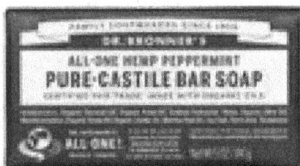

Ingredients to avoid:
PEG, Ceteareth, polyethylene, parabens, DMDM Hydantoin

Pono choice:
Puna Noni Naturals

Why we love it:
Ingredients that will love your hair and vice versa, coupled with large bottles for bulk refilling at the store means that Puna Noni will give you great hair and a cleaner conscience.

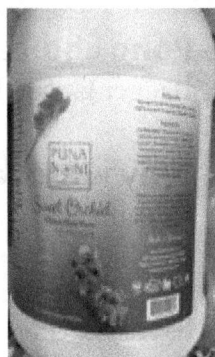

Soap

Ingredients to avoid:
Triclosan, Triclocarban, 1-4 dioxane, Bronopol

Pono choice:
Dr. Bronner's Pure Castile Bar Soap

Why we love it:
In addition to being a global leader in sustainability, the Bronners family brand produces products with minimal packaging and great ingredients.

Hand Cleanser/Sanitizer

Ingredients to avoid:
Triclosan, and anything you can't easily pronounce!

Pono choice:
Everyone Hand Sanitizing Spray

Why we love it:
Compare the ingredients in this spray to the CleanWell foaming rub, and you'll see that this sanitizer has all ingredients easy to pronounce...a fairly reliable guide when you're in doubt. The aluminum container reduces plastic waste and is recyclable. Everyone is a certified B-corporation, meaning their company does a lot of good things. There's a lot of applications of sanitizer in this little bottle, too, meaning a lot less cost, and much less waste than hand wipes!

Sunscreen

Ingredients to avoid:
Oxybenzone, Benzalkonium, retinyl palmitate, retinol

Pono choice:
Little Hands Hawaii

Why we love it:
A zinc oxide topical sunscreen with a balance of great ingredients. Reef safe, kiddie safe, hypoallergenic, and comes in a plastic-free, 100% recyclable aluminum tin.

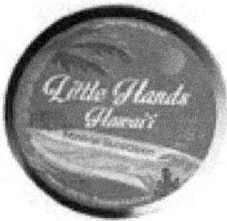

Insect Repellent

Ingredients to avoid:
DEET

Pono choice:
Badger Anti-Bug Balm

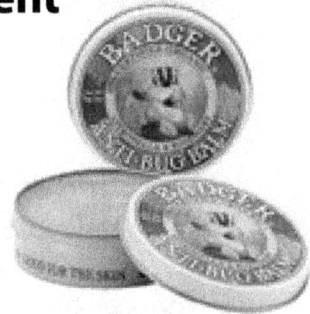

Why we love it:
A delightful smelling balm that you can spread onto any exposed skin, the Badger Anti-Bug Balm contains mostly citronella, rosemary, and other natural scents that bugs typically steer clear of.

If you prefer a spray, Badger has a great bug spray with a much higher proportion of citronella than the Burt's Bees version, meaning more insect repelling per dollar spent.

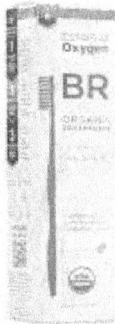

Toothpaste

Ingredients to avoid:
Triclosan

Pono choice:
BR Organic Toothpaste

Why we love it:
Food-grade hydrogen peroxide cleanses, whitens, and disinfects your teeth, and then biodegrades into water and pure oxygen. The balance of the ingredients are relatively healthy thickeners and essential oils with a variety of benefits for your teeth and gums.

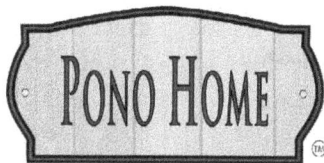

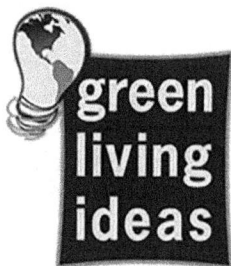

Pono Home and the *Green Living Ideas* book are based upon work supported by the Department of Energy, the Department of Defense, and the Office of Naval Research, who have all funded the Elemental Excelerator. Any reports from Pono Home were prepared as an account of work sponsored by an agency of the United States government. Neither the U.S. government nor any agency thereof, nor any of their employees, makes any warranty, express or implied, or assumes any legal liability or responsibility for the accuracy, completeness, or usefulness of any information, apparatus, product or process disclosed, or represents that its use would not infringe privately owned rights. Reference herein to any specific commercial product, process, or service by trade name, trademark, manufacturer, or otherwise does not necessarily constitute or imply its endorsement, recommendation, or favoring by the U.S. government or any agency thereof. The views and opinions of authors expressed herein do not necessarily state or reflect those of the U.S. government or any agency thereof.

Glossary

chemical burden
Buildup of synthetic chemicals and heavy metals in our bodies over time, which can produce negative health effects.

eco-driving
The practice of driving to minimize fuel consumption and the emission of carbon dioxide.

GMO
Genetically modified organism: an organism or micro-organism that has had its DNA altered via genetic engineering.

off-gassing
The emission of noxious gases.

PERC
Perchloroethylene: a chemical used for dry cleaning, which can evaporate into indoor air and has been linked to some cancers.

petrochemical
A chemical substance obtained from petroleum or natural gas.

pono
Hawaiian word commonly translated as "righteousness."

PSI
Pounds per square inch: a measure of tire pressure.

References Cited

i. http://cleantechnica.com/2014/11/20/germanys-renewable-energy-market-charts/
ii. *Unlocking Energy Efficiency in the US Economy.* McKinsey and Company. July 2009. http://bit.ly/jxtVb4
iii. http://www.imt.org/news/the-current/owners-of-efficient-homes-less-likely-to-default
iv. http://www.ncbi.nlm.nih.gov/pmc/articles/PMC1651599/
v. http://eatdrinkbetter.com/2014/10/21/the-china-study-campbell-nutrition/
vi. http://www.nrdc.org/food/files/wasted-food-ip.pdf
vii. http://www.epa.gov/osw/conserve/materials/plastics.htm
viii. http://www.fueleconomy.gov/feg/maintain.shtml
ix. *The Non-Toxic Avenger.* Deanna Duke.

Artwork Credits

Start a business to save the world?

Have you ever wanted to have a job that makes a positive difference in the world? Wouldn't it be great if, every day, you saw the fruits of your labor, made peoples' lives better, and made a living doing so? And wouldn't it be even better if instead of just a job doing this, you could own and build a business doing this?

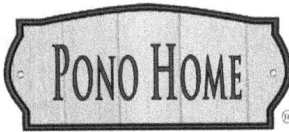

Pono Home may just be the answer for you. Pono Home is a green home service that brings sustainability into the home in a convenient, efficient, and effective way. Pono Home professionals enter a home and by the time they leave, they can cut energy use by 25% and water use by 30%! Imagine the positive impacts you'll have on the environment, on peoples' lives, and in your community. The company is planning to franchise operations starting in 2018, and is looking to help people like you build a powerful business that will change the world, one home at a time.

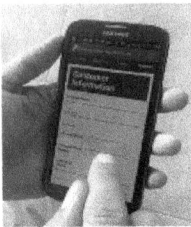

Our proprietary mobile software will guide you through home services, making your job easy and efficient. Record-keeping, report generating, inventory tracking, accounting, and revenue generation are all built in!

You like tools? Pono Home services are conducted with the latest and greatest sustainability auditing tools. We train you to use them, and keep you up to date when new technology emerges.

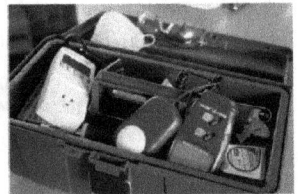

Pono Home was founded by the author of this book, Scott Cooney, in 2013 with the mission of helping people live healthier, greener lives, for life.

To find out if you're a good candidate for becoming a Pono Home franchisee, visit http://bit.ly/12T7D0l to take a franchisee quiz. Also, please visit our website, at www.PonoHome.com.

What customers are saying about Pono Home:

"Frankly, this might be the best deal going. Everyone should look into having Pono Home do a service. You will earn back the cost (already very reasonable) pretty quickly with a lower utility bill. Can't recommend this company more highly."

— Kate M.

"After watching the Pono Home service, I am now a lot more aware of where my electricity is being used unnecessarily. Both at work and at home, now, we can start saving money and energy right away. Thank you...very much, Pono Home!"

— Scott Williams, President, Lex Brodie's

"Pono Home made it easy for me to be healthier and greener. I found it so refreshing to have non-judgmental, knowledgeable pros come in and green my home. With their service and this book, Pono Home makes greening your home as easy as 1-2-3..."

— Dawn Lippert, CEO, Elemental Excelerator

"Pono Home is a wonderful service! You would not believe how much energy and water you can save until you have this team come and fix your house. Not only do LED lights use less power, but they are even brighter...I highly recommend you call them today and watch your energy and water bill drop!"

— Greg M.